LOW OXALATE
DIET COOKBOOK AND FOOD LIST FOR SENIORS

A Complete Guide with Healthy Recipes and A 30-Day Meal Plan to Manage Kidney Stone

HILDA M. JACOBS

Copyright © 2024 by Hilda M. Jacobs

All rights reserved.
No part of this publication may be reproduced, distributed, or transmitted in any form or by any means, including photocopying, recording, or other electronic or mechanical methods, without the prior written permission of the publisher, except in the case of brief quotations embodied in critical reviews and certain other noncommercial uses permitted by copyright law.

Disclaimer: The information provided in this book, is intended for educational purposes only. It is not a substitute for professional medical advice, diagnosis, or treatment. Always seek the advice of your physician or other qualified healthcare provider with any questions you may have regarding a medical condition.

The author and publisher of this book have made every effort to ensure that the information provided is accurate and up-to-date at the time of publication. However, medical knowledge and research are constantly evolving, and information may become outdated or subject to change. Therefore, the author and publisher do not warrant or guarantee the accuracy, completeness, or timeliness of the information presented in this book.
The author and publisher shall not be liable for any direct or indirect damages or injuries arising out of the use, interpretation, or application of any information provided in this book. Readers are encouraged to consult with their healthcare providers for individualized advice and recommendations based on their specific medical conditions and needs. By reading this book, you acknowledge and agree to the terms of this disclaimer.

Printed in the United States of America.

First Edition: April 202

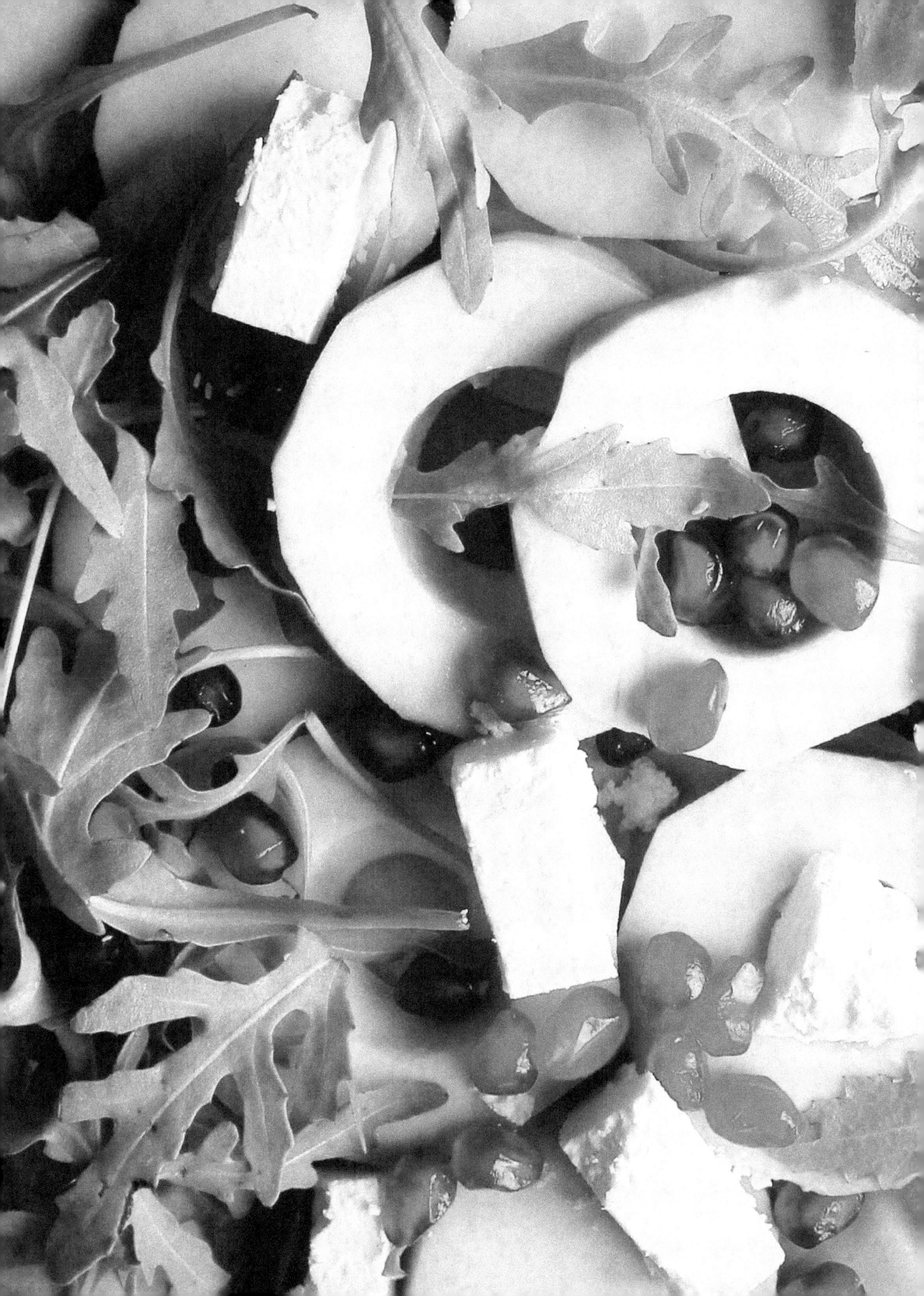

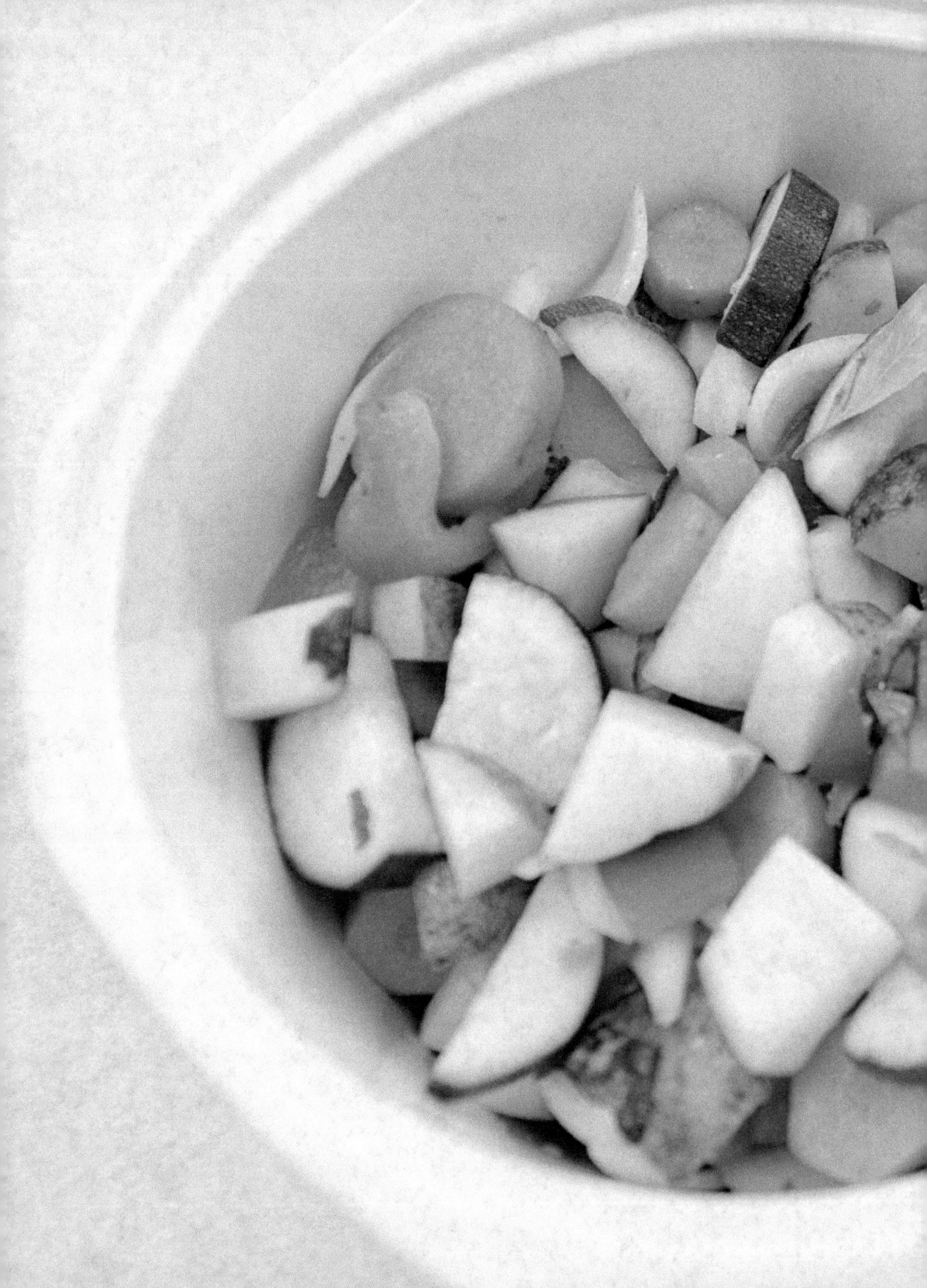

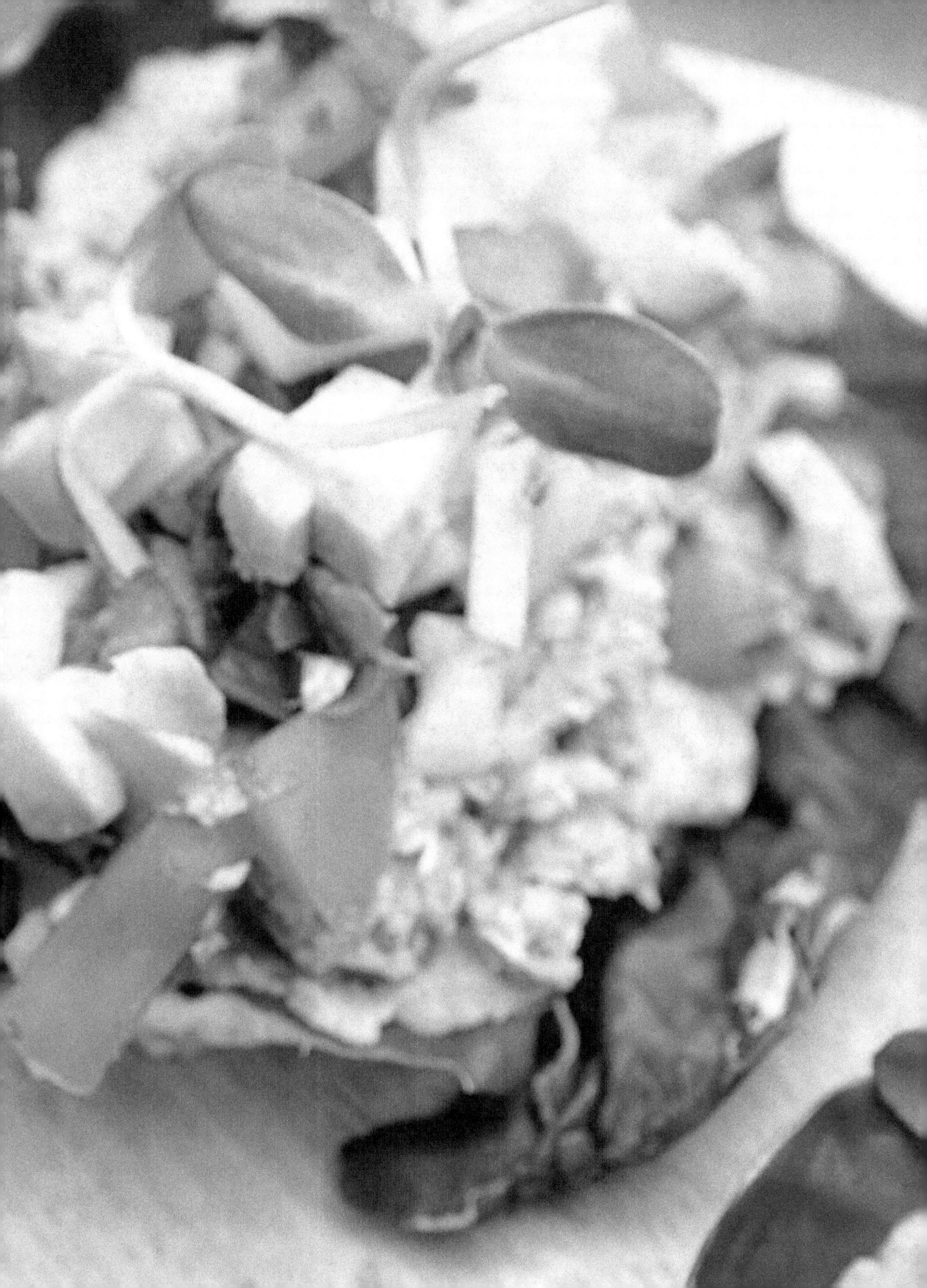

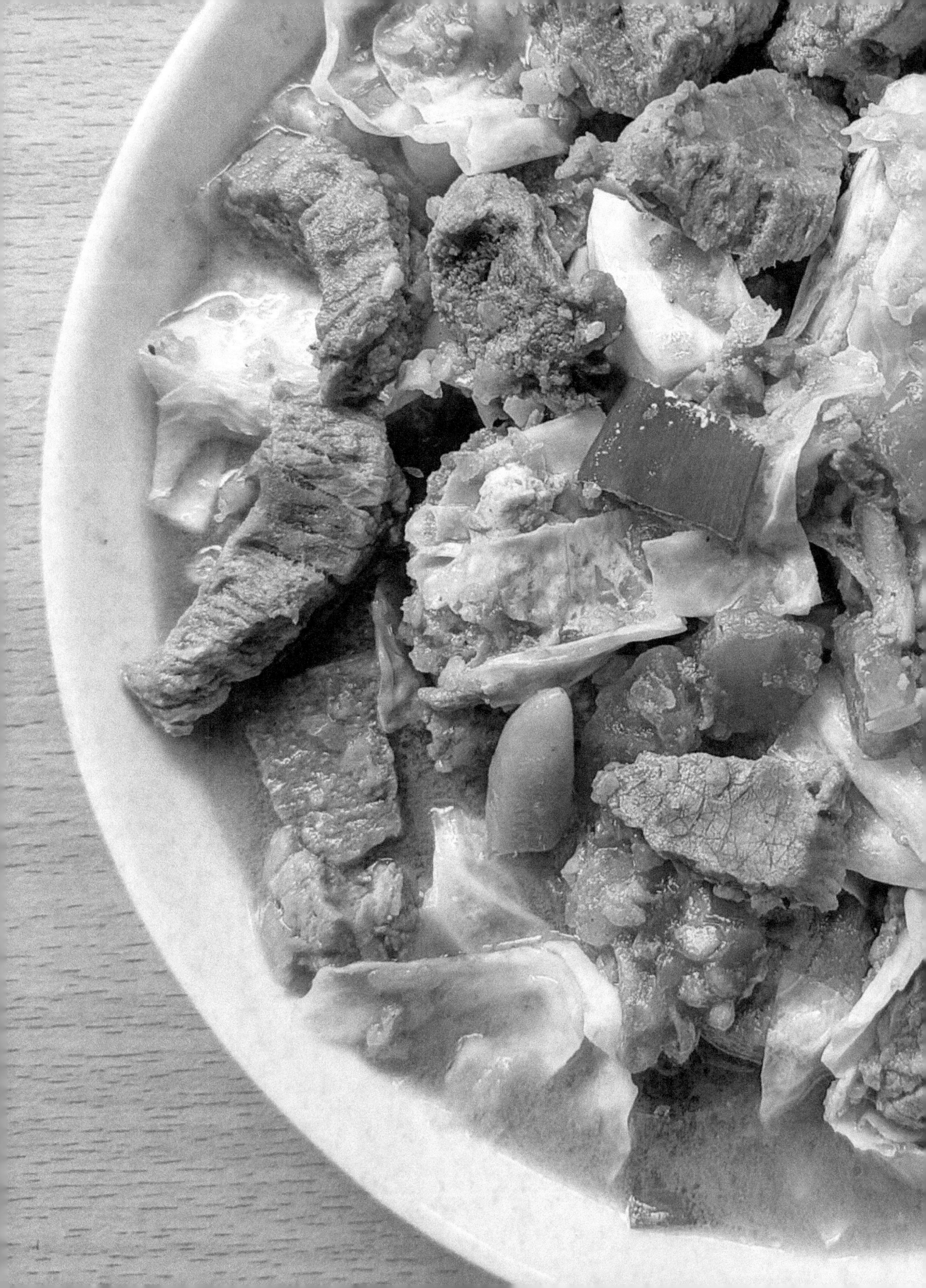

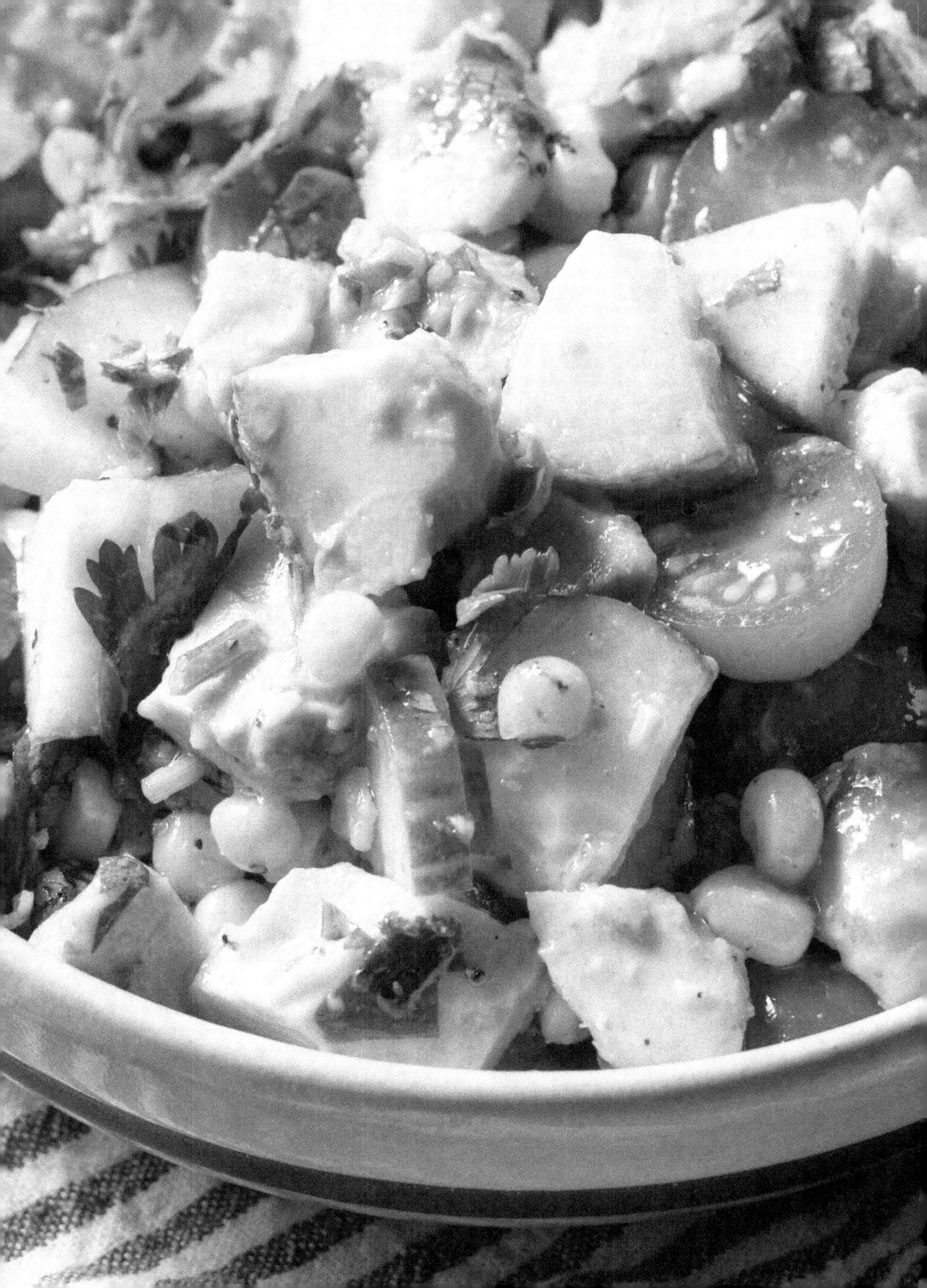

CONTENTS

INTRODUCTION 1

UNDERSTANDING OXALATES 3

    Oxalates: A Comprehensive Overview 3

    Impact of Oxalates on the Body 4

    Symptoms of High Oxalate 5

    Diagnostic Approaches for Oxalate Levels 6

    Worksheet: Understanding Oxalates 6

BENEFITS OF A LOW OXALATE DIET 11

    Worksheet: Benefits of a Low Oxalate Diet 13

FOOD LISTS FOR LOW OXALATE 18

    Vegetables 18

    Fruits 20

    Grain/Cereal 21

    Nuts and Seeds 22

    Legumes 24

    Herbs and Spices 26

BREAKFAST RECIPES 28

    Oatmeal with Fresh Berries and Almonds 28

    Scrambled Eggs with Spinach and Feta 28

    Avocado Toast with Poached Egg 29

    Cottage Cheese and Pineapple Bowl 30

    Quinoa Breakfast Porridge 30

    Baked Avocado Eggs 31

Greek Yogurt with Mixed Nuts and Honey 31

Chia Seed Pudding with Kiwi 32

Quinoa Breakfast Bowl 32

Berry Smoothie with Spinach 33

MAIN DISH RECIPES 33

Grilled Chicken with Herb Salad 33

Baked Salmon with Asparagus 34

Quinoa Stuffed Bell Peppers 34

Turkey and Vegetable Skillet 34

Lentil Soup with Spinach 35

Baked Cod with Roasted Vegetables 36

Turkey Meatballs in Tomato Sauce 36

Grilled Vegetable Platter 37

Cauliflower Steak with Herb Sauce 38

Baked Tilapia with Lemon and Dill 38

SNACKS RECIPES 40

Cucumber and Hummus Bites 40

Apple Slices with Almond Butter 40

Greek Yogurt with Honey and Walnuts 41

Carrot Sticks with Avocado Dip 41

Baked Kale Chips 42

Roasted Chickpeas 42

Zucchini Chips 43

Peanut Butter Banana Bites 43

Cucumber Roll-Ups with Hummus 44

Avocado Toast with Cherry Tomatoes 44

VEGETABLES AND SALAD 45

Mixed Greens with Apple and Walnuts ....45.

Cucumber Tomato Salad 45

Roasted Beet and Goat Cheese Salad 46

Carrot Slaw with Cranberries 46

Spinach and Strawberry Salad 47

Avocado and Tomato Salad 48

Broccoli and Cauliflower Salad 48

Cucumber Dill Salad 49

Mixed Bean Salad 49

Shaved Brussels Sprout Salad 50

SOUP AND STEW 51

Chicken and Rice Soup 51

Tomato Basil Soup 51

Lentil Vegetable Stew 52

Butternut Squash Soup 53

Carrot Ginger Soup 53

Zucchini Basil Soup 54

Creamy Mushroom Soup 55

Sweet Potato and Lentil Stew 55

Creamy Cauliflower Soup 56

Chicken Vegetable Soup 56

DESSERT RECIPES 58

Baked Apples with Cinnamon 58

Vanilla Rice Pudding 58

Peach Yogurt Parfait 59

Berry Gelatin Cups 59

Coconut Mango Mousse 60

Almond and Berry Crumble 60

Lemon Ricotta Cake 61

Chocolate Avocado Pudding 61

No-Bake Coconut Balls 62

Baked Peach Crisp 62

SMOOTHIE RECIPES 64

Blueberry Almond Smoothie 64

Spinach Avocado Smoothie 64

Strawberry Oatmeal Breakfast Smoothie 65

Carrot Ginger Turmeric Smoothie 65

Mango Coconut Water Smoothie 66

Banana Almond Smoothie 66

Blueberry Spinach Smoothie 67

Strawberry Cucumber Smoothie 67

Peach Ginger Smoothie 68

Carrot Apple Ginger Smoothie 68

30-DAY MEAL PLAN 69

INTERACTIVE TOOLS 76

Oxalate Food Diary 76

Oxalate Symptom Tracker 78

Meal Planning Guide 80

Hydration Tracker 83

Medication and Supplement Monitor 85

- Recipe Modification Worksheet 88
- Nutrient Intake Chart 91
- Eating Out Guide: Low-Oxalate Choices 93
- Progress Reflection and Goal Setting Sheets 95

CONCLUSION 98

INTRODUCTION

Here I am, nestled in my favorite chair, tea in hand, watching the rain paint the streets of New York with its soft, rhythmic strokes. It's a day for woolen socks, for reflection, a day that whispers of stories untold. Among these, one story beats vividly in my heart - the saga of my Aunt Martha. At the ripe age of 79, she unfolded before me lessons of life, resilience, and the courage to embrace change, lessons that no one else has ever etched so deeply into my soul.

Aunt Martha, with her New York abode that buzzed with the energy of endless social gatherings, was more than just family. Her home was a sanctuary where the scent of freshly baked cakes lingered, and laughter about her latest garden misadventure was never far off. But a shadow fell over this warmth about a year ago when Aunt Martha began to feel the weight of her years. Fatigue, aching joints, and a discomfort she waved off as the toll of time became her constant companions.

Her concerns led her to Dr. Charlie, the family doctor who had seen her through decades of vibrancy. The diagnosis caught us off guard - a battle against high oxalates in her body, threatening her with kidney stones. I can still hear her voice, laced with disbelief, over the phone, "Oxalates, can you believe it? Those tiny things in my beloved spinach and chocolate."

But Aunt Martha, ever the fighter, refused to let this challenge dictate her sunset years. She faced her new dietary restrictions head-on, with a spirit that would put many to shame. It was a daunting task, to change one's diet so drastically at 79, yet she met it with a determination that was nothing short of inspiring.

Her kitchen turned into a playground for culinary experimentation. Sundays became our tasting days, where she'd serve up her latest creations, like her roasted carrot and quinoa salad, eyes gleaming with the excitement of a child. It was a journey of hits and misses, but through it, her cacao nib cookies emerged victorious, a testament to her enduring spirit.

More than her diet changed; Aunt Martha embraced a lifestyle transformation. Yoga, once as alien to her as the concept of jumping out of a plane, became her new passion. She'd joke about out-bending her younger self, her laughter filling the room with light.

Watching her, an idea began to take root in my mind. Aunt Martha's journey, her battles, and victories, carried a wealth of wisdom that could inspire countless others, especially seniors navigating their own health challenges. With a background in nutrition, I'd always focused on broad dietary guidelines, but here was a narrative that delved into the often-overlooked nuances of managing oxalates in one's diet.

Thus was born the idea for "Low Oxalate Diet Cookbook, Meal Plan, and Food List for Seniors." This book wasn't to be just another dietary guide; it was to be a conversation, an intimate sharing of Aunt Martha's journey interwoven with professional insights.

In writing this book, Aunt Martha's insights were invaluable, her stories and experiences lending authenticity and depth. Our discussions, the stories from her blog, and our kitchen experiments became the soul of this project.

A year into this new chapter, the transformation in Aunt Martha was undeniable. Her energy, her zest for life, was palpable. The project thrilled her, and when Dr. Charlie confirmed the drop in her oxalate levels, her laughter was triumphant. She wasn't just the muse for the book; she was its first victory.

The book is a tapestry of Aunt Martha's journey - from the initial struggles to the joy of overcoming them. It's packed with practical advice, recipes that don't feel like sacrifices, and tips to make this daunting change more manageable for seniors. But beyond that, it's a narrative of community, of the pivotal role of support and understanding in navigating the path to better health.

As I sit here, manuscript in hand, the journey feels full circle. This book, borne of Aunt Martha's resilience and her unwavering spirit, has not only enriched my professional insights but has profoundly touched my heart. It's a testament to the power of change, to the endless potential within us to adapt and thrive, regardless of age. With my tea cooling beside me, I can't help but feel an overwhelming sense of gratitude for the incredible journey Aunt Martha and I have shared. It's a story of love, of learning, and, ultimately, of living fully, no matter the obstacles we face.

UNDERSTANDING OXALATES

Oxalates: A Comprehensive Overview

In nutrition and health, the concept of oxalates emerges as a significant subject that frequently piques interest and sometimes prompts concerns. These organic compounds, prevalent across a diverse range of foods—from the verdant leaves adorning our dishes to the sturdy beans forming the core of our meals—play a crucial role within the natural cycles of plant, animal, and human life, impacting our dietary practices and overall health.

Oxalates, by their nature, are known for their propensity to bind with minerals, notably calcium, creating formations that may pose challenges for absorption within the human body. This characteristic interaction highlights the need for mindful consumption, especially for individuals dealing with specific health conditions like kidney stones, where oxalate management is integral to dietary planning.

The journey of oxalates through our digestive tract involves a complex interplay with minerals, potentially leading to crystal formations that, in excess, can precipitate the development of kidney stones— a condition characterized by significant discomfort and prevalent among a considerable segment of the population. While most people can process oxalates with efficiency, courtesy of our kidneys' regulatory functions, individuals with particular health considerations might require a more nuanced understanding of oxalate intake to make strategic dietary decisions.

Exploring the topic of oxalates invites us to reevaluate our dietary choices, encouraging us to view our meals not merely as nourishment or pleasure but as integral parts of a broader health narrative. Each morsel we consume carries implications for how it interacts with our physiology and contributes to our overall well-being.

Beyond the scientific aspect, understanding oxalates encourages a deeper connection with our dietary habits, prompting reflections on our relationship with food, our bodies, and the health decisions we face each day. It underlines the importance of considering our food choices as expressions of self-care, armed with the knowledge necessary to align our diet with our health objectives.

Impact of Oxalates on the Body

The relationship between oxalates and human health is diverse, impacting individuals differently based on their health status. For many, oxalates are harmlessly excreted from the body, yet for those with specific health conditions, elevated oxalate levels pose a significant risk, leading to a variety of medical complications. It is essential to grasp the influence of oxalates on human health to effectively manage their effects and safeguard one's well-being.

Kidney Stones: The primary concern with high oxalate concentration is its contribution to the formation of kidney stones. Oxalates can combine with calcium in the urine, forming calcium oxalate stones. These stones can cluster, obstructing urine flow and causing excruciating pain, potentially culminating in kidney damage if not addressed. Individuals with a predisposition to kidney stones are often counseled to moderate their consumption of foods high in oxalates, mitigating the risk of stone development.

Bone Health: Emerging research indicates a potential link between oxalates and bone health, particularly in older adults or those with concerns about bone density. Oxalates may hinder calcium absorption by binding to it in the digestive system, thus limiting the calcium available for bolstering bone strength and density. This can be particularly detrimental for those at increased risk of osteoporosis.

Gastrointestinal Health: A diet rich in oxalates can also adversely affect gastrointestinal wellness. Ingesting substantial amounts of oxalates may irritate the digestive tract, manifesting as abdominal discomfort, bloating, and diarrhea. This poses an additional challenge for those with pre-existing conditions such as inflammatory bowel disease or irritable bowel syndrome, who may find their symptoms exacerbated by high oxalate intake.

Nutrient Absorption: Oxalates in the digestive tract can disrupt the absorption of critical minerals, including calcium, magnesium, and iron, by binding to them. This interference can lead to deficiencies, adversely affecting overall health. These minerals are integral to various physiological functions, including immune defense, muscle operation, and neural communication.

Oxalate Sensitivity and Hyperoxaluria: Certain individuals exhibit an increased sensitivity to oxalates or suffer from hyperoxaluria, a condition characterized by the body's excessive production or absorption of oxalates. Whether genetic (primary) or caused by diet, gut health, or other medical conditions (secondary), this sensitivity can precipitate serious health issues such as kidney stones and compromised bone health even with standard dietary oxalate levels.

Gut Microbiome's Influence: The gut microbiome significantly affects oxalate processing in the body. Some gut bacteria can degrade oxalates, diminishing their absorption and subsequent accumulation in the body. A disruption in the balance of these beneficial bacteria can increase oxalate absorption, underscoring the crucial role of maintaining gut health for regulating oxalate levels and promoting overall health.

Symptoms of High Oxalate

Elevated oxalate concentrations, a medical condition termed hyperoxaluria, can provoke a spectrum of symptoms and complications, with a significant impact on the kidneys and urinary system. The presence of oxalate crystals in the body can lead to various health concerns, detailed below:

1. **Kidney Stones**: The formation of calcium oxalate stones is a notable result of elevated oxalate levels, presenting symptoms such as intense pain in the back, sides, abdomen, or groin, the appearance of blood in the urine, increased urination frequency, pain during urination, and nausea.
2. **Urinary Tract Complications**: The urinary tract may become irritated, manifesting in increased urination frequency, discomfort during urination, and cloudy urine.
3. **Kidney Damage**: Persistent high oxalate levels can cause chronic kidney disease, marked by diminished kidney function, swelling due to fluid retention, fatigue, cognitive difficulties, and reduced urine production.
4. **Digestive System Effects**: High dietary oxalate intake or compromised gut health can cause abdominal discomfort, diarrhea, bloating, and gas. In cases of gut disorders, nutrient absorption may be impaired.
5. **Bone and Joint Pain**: In rare instances, such as with primary hyperoxaluria, oxalate crystals can accumulate in bones and joints, leading to pain, stiffness, and reduced mobility.
6. **Skin Conditions**: Oxalate deposits in the skin can cause itchiness, irritation, and rashes.
7. **Vulvar Pain**: For women, elevated oxalate levels might result in vulvar discomfort or vulvodynia.
8. **Systemic Oxalosis**: In severe cases, oxalate accumulation can affect multiple organs, leading to broad complications.

It is crucial to understand that these symptoms can be indicative of various health issues. Accurate medical evaluation and diagnosis are essential for anyone experiencing such symptoms or suspecting high oxalate levels.

Diagnostic Approaches for Oxalate Levels

1. **Urine Analysis**: A primary method for assessing oxalate levels involves urine tests. These include:
   - **24-Hour Urine Collection**: This comprehensive approach requires collecting all urine within 24 hours to analyze oxalate levels, offering insight into daily fluctuations and other risk factors for stone formation.
   - **Spot Urine Testing**: This method analyzes a single sample to provide a snapshot of oxalate levels at a specific time, though it may not accurately reflect daily variations.
2. **Blood Tests**: Although less common, blood tests can measure oxalate levels, offering insights into oxalate metabolism and potential health impacts. Factors such as hydration and diet can affect these readings, requiring careful interpretation.
3. **Tissue Biopsy**: In specific, severe cases, particularly for diagnosing genetic conditions leading to oxalate accumulation, a tissue biopsy might be conducted.
4. **Genetic Testing**: For suspected genetic conditions affecting oxalate metabolism, such as primary hyperoxaluria, genetic testing can identify mutations, aiding in treatment and management strategies.

Worksheet: Understanding Oxalates

Section 1: What are Oxalates?

Definition: Oxalates are organic compounds found in many types of food, and they can also be produced as waste products by the body. Write a short note on how you think oxalates affect the body based on your prior knowledge:

_____

_____

_____

_____

_____

Section 2: Sources of Oxalates

Table 1: Common Foods High in Oxalates

Complete the table with the oxalate content rating (High, Medium, Low) based on what you've learned or researched.

Food Item	Oxalate Content Rating
Spinach	
Chocolate	
Almonds	
Beets	
Potatoes	

Section 3: Health Implications of High Oxalate Levels

Key Points: High levels of oxalates can lead to health issues such as kidney stones, urinary tract problems, and more. In the lines below, summarize why managing oxalate intake might be important for individuals with certain health conditions:

_____

_____

_____

_____

_____

_____

_____

_____

Section 4: Identifying Symptoms of High Oxalate Levels
- **Checklist**: Mark the symptoms that are commonly associated with high oxalate levels.
    - ☐ Kidney Stones
    - ☐ Frequent Urination
    - ☐ Bone Pain
    - ☐ Muscle Weakness
    - ☐ Abdominal Pain
    - ☐ Itchy Skin

Section 5: Management and Prevention

Strategies: List some strategies that can help manage or reduce oxalate levels in the body. Use the lines below for your answers.

_____

_____

_____

_____

_____

Section 6: Testing for Oxalate Levels

Discussion: Why is it important to test for oxalate levels, and what methods can be used? Reflect on the reasons for testing and list at least two methods described earlier in the worksheet.

_____

_____

_____

_____

_____

Section 7: Reflection and Personal Application

Questions: Based on what you've learned, how might you apply this knowledge to your diet or lifestyle? Are there any changes you would consider making?

_____

_____

_____

_____

_____

Section 8: Further Research

Prompt: Choose a topic related to oxalates that interests you for further research. It could be a deep dive into oxalate metabolism, the role of the gut microbiome in oxalate processing, or exploring low-oxalate diets. Outline your research question or objective:

_____

_____

_____

_____

_____

BENEFITS OF A LOW OXALATE DIET

Adopting a diet low in oxalates, though aimed primarily at reducing oxalate consumption, offers a wide spectrum of advantages, especially for those with specific health concerns or dietary restrictions.

1. **Minimized Risk of Kidney Stones**: Primarily beneficial for individuals prone to forming kidney stones, especially those comprised of calcium oxalate. Diminishing oxalate intake can drastically reduce the likelihood of stone development, a critical consideration for anyone with a history of kidney stones due to their increased risk of recurrence.
2. **Enhanced Mineral Absorption**: Oxalates can hinder the absorption of crucial minerals such as calcium and magnesium, essential for a host of bodily functions. A reduction in oxalate consumption can thus enhance the uptake and bioavailability of these minerals, supporting bone health. This is of particular importance to postmenopausal women and the elderly, who are at a heightened risk of osteoporosis.
3. **Improved Digestive Wellness**: By limiting potential dietary irritants, a low oxalate regimen can contribute to better digestive health. This is notably advantageous for those suffering from gastrointestinal issues, such as irritable bowel syndrome (IBS) or inflammatory bowel disease (IBD), where minimizing dietary triggers can alleviate symptoms and enhance life quality.
4. **Alleviation of Oxalate-Linked Discomfort**: In conditions like vulvodynia, characterized by chronic vulvar pain, some research has indicated a correlation with elevated oxalate levels. Reports from patients adhering to a low oxalate diet often include significant pain reduction, hinting at a possible connection between dietary oxalates and symptom intensity in such conditions.
5. **Enhanced Management of Chronic Health Issues**: For those dealing with long-term health problems, integrating a low oxalate diet with other dietary and therapeutic measures can be particularly effective. This approach is especially pertinent for chronic kidney disease management, where oxalate regulation is crucial for preserving kidney function.
6. **Possible Decrease in Inflammation**: While further investigation is needed to fully elucidate the relationship between oxalates and inflammation, preliminary evidence suggests that high dietary oxalate levels may exacerbate inflammatory responses. Consequently, a diet lower in oxalates might

aid in diminishing systemic inflammation, offering relief from conditions such as arthritis and other inflammatory disorders.

7. **Elevated Overall Dietary Quality**: Focusing on reducing oxalate intake generally encourages a comprehensive dietary approach, leading to the adoption of healthier eating patterns. This includes a broader inclusion of low oxalate fruits, vegetables, grains, and lean proteins, thereby enhancing nutritional intake and overall health.

8. **Encouragement of Hydration and Health-Conscious Lifestyle Choices**: The management of oxalate levels often comes with advice to maintain optimal hydration, aiding in the elimination of excess oxalates. This focus on fluid intake can yield further health benefits, such as improved kidney function and general physical well-being. Additionally, pursuing a low oxalate diet can motivate broader healthy lifestyle decisions, including regular physical activity and moderation in the consumption of alcohol and caffeine.

9. **Personalization According to Individual Requirements**: A low oxalate diet allows for customization to meet personal dietary preferences and needs, making it both effective and sustainable over time. It empowers individuals to engage actively with their dietary choices, fostering a greater understanding of the impact of nutrition on health.

Worksheet: Benefits of a Low Oxalate Diet

Section 1: Health Benefits

Complete the table below by listing the health benefits of reducing oxalate intake, based on the information provided or your own research.

Benefit	Description (How it helps)	Personal Importance (High/Medium/Low)
Reduced Risk of Kidney Stones		
Enhanced Mineral Absorption		
Improved Digestive Health		
Alleviation of Oxalate-Linked Discomfort		
Better Chronic Condition Management		
Potential Reduction in Inflammation		
Improved Overall Dietary Quality		
Promotes Hydration and Healthy Lifestyles		
Customization to Individual Dietary Needs		

Section 2: Symptom Tracker

Before starting a low oxalate diet, track any current symptoms you experience that may be related to high oxalate intake.

Symptom

_____

_____

_____

_____

Frequency

_____

_____

_____

_____

Severity

_____

_____

_____

_____

_____

Section 3: Diet Planning

Plan a day's menu that aligns with a low oxalate diet. Include options for breakfast, lunch, dinner, and snacks. Consider incorporating foods that are both low in oxalates and high in nutritional value.

Breakfast

_____

_____

_____

_____

Lunch

_____

_____

_____

_____

Dinner

_____

_____

_____

_____

Snacks

_____

_____

Section 4: Lifestyle Adjustments

Beyond diet, list any lifestyle changes you can make to support a low oxalate diet and improve your overall health.

_____

_____

_____

_____

Section 5: Goal Setting

Set specific, measurable goals for implementing a low oxalate diet into your life. Consider short-term and long-term objectives.

Short-term goal

_____

_____

_____

_____

Long-term goal

_____

_____

_____

_____

Section 7: Reflective Notes

After reviewing the benefits and planning steps, reflect on how a low oxalate diet might impact your health and lifestyle.

_____

_____

_____

_____

FOOD LISTS FOR LOW OXALATE

Vegetables

Vegetable	Portion Size	Oxalate (mg)	Calories	Protein (g)	Fiber (g)
Acorn Squash	1 cup (205g)	1	57	2.1	10
Artichoke	1 medium	16	61	5.2	7.9
Arugula	1 cup (20g)	2	6	1.5	1.6
Asparagus	1 cup (134g)	4	28	3.9	3.8
Bamboo Shoots	1 cup (151g)	2	14	3	3.2
Bell Pepper	1 medium	6	25	2	2.5
Bitter Melon	1 cup (124g)	1	17	2	3.6
Black Olives	1 cup (135g)	11	156	2.2	4.3
Bok Choy	1 cup (70g)	2	10	2	2
Butternut Squash	1 cup (205g)	3	83	2.8	7.6
Cabbage	1 cup (89g)	21	23	2	3.2
Celery	1 cup (101g)	6	17	1.7	2.6
Collard Greens	1 cup (36g)	6	12	2	2.4
Eggplant	1 cup (99g)	4	21	1.8	3.5
Endive	1 cup (50g)	3	10	1.6	2.8
Fennel Bulb	1 cup (87g)	5	28	2	3.7
Garlic	1 clove (3g)	2	5	1.2	1.1
Ginger	1 tsp (2g)	2	3	1.04	1
Green Beans	1 cup (125g)	38	32	2.8	4.4

Jalapeno Peppers	1 pepper (14g)	1	5	1.2	1.4
Jicama	1 cup (130g)	4	47	1.9	7.4
Kohlrabi	1 cup (135g)	1	37	3.3	5.9
Leeks	1 cup (89g)	90	55	2.3	2.6
Lettuce	1 cup (47g)	1	6	1.5	1.5
Mustard Greens	1 cup (56g)	5	16	2.5	2.8
Onion	1 cup (160g)	14	65	2.8	3.7
Parsnips	1 cup (133g)	11	101	2.6	7.5
Pumpkin	1 cup (116g)	3	31	2.2	1.6
Radicchio	1 cup (40g)	1	10	1.6	1.9
Radishes	1 cup (116g)	3	20	1.8	2.9
Rutabaga	1 cup (140g)	1	53	2.5	4.2
Snow Peas	1 cup (98g)	1	36	3.8	3.6
Sweet Potato	1 cup (200g)	29	181	5	7.6
Tomato	1 medium	6	23	2.1	2.5
Turnips	1 cup (130g)	20	37	2.2	4.1
Watercress	1 cup (34g)	1.8	5	1.8	1.2
Wax Beans	1 cup (110g)	1	35	2.8	4.6
Yellow Squash	1 cup (113g)	5	19	2.4	2.2

Fruits

Fruits	Portion Size	Oxalate (mg)	Calories	Carbs (g)	Protein (g)	Fiber (g)
Apple	1 medium	3	96	25	5	20
Banana	1 medium	4	106	27	4	15
Orange	1 medium	1	63	15	4	13
Strawberry	1 cup (152g)	3	50	12	4	8
Blueberry	1 cup (148g)	5	85	21	5	16
Watermelon	1 cup (152g)	1	47	12	2	10
Peach	1 medium	2	60	14	3	14
Pineapple	1 cup (165g)	3	83	22	3	17
Grapes	1 cup (151g)	6	105	27	2	24
Kiwi	1 medium	3	43	10	3	7
Mango	1 cup (165g)	3	100	25	4	24
Cherries	1 cup (138g)	4	88	22	4	18
Pomegranate	1 cup (174g)	6	145	32	8	25
Pear	1 medium	5	102	27	7	18
Blackberries	1 cup (144g)	5	63	14	9	8
Raspberries	1 cup (123g)	5	65	15	9	6
Cantaloupe	1 cup (160g)	1	54	13	2	13
Papaya	1 cup (145g)	3	63	16	4	12
Lemon	1 medium	2	18	5	3	2
Lime	1 medium	3	21	7	3	2
Avocado	1 cup (150g)	3	241	13	11	2
Fig	1 medium	3	38	10	3	9
Plum	1 medium	2	31	8	2	8
Nectarine	1 medium	1	64	15	3	12

Honeydew Melon	1 cup (170g)	1	65	16	2	15
Apricot	1 medium	2	18	4	2	4
Guava	1 medium	3	39	8	4	6
Persimmon	1 medium	3	119	31	7	22
Tangerine	1 medium	3	48	12	3	10
Cranberries	1 cup (100g)	7	47	12	5	5

Grain/Cereal

Grain/Cereal	Portion Size	Oxalate (mg)	Calories	Carbs (g)	Protein (g)	Fiber (g)
Barley Flakes	1 cup (40g)	7	145	33	5	9
Bran Flakes	1 cup (29g)	6	99	25	4	6
Chia Seeds	1 oz (28g)	3	138	13	5.4	11.6
Corn Flakes	1 cup (28g)	2	102	25	2.9	1.9
Couscous	1 cup (157g)	6	177	37	7	3.2
Cream of Wheat	1 cup (251g)	2	127	28	4.6	2.3
Flaxseeds	1 tbsp (10g)	8	56	4	2.9	3.8
Granola	1 cup (122g)	5	598	65	19	12
Hemp Seeds	1 tbsp (30g)	4	167	3.6	10.5	2.2
Instant Oatmeal	1 packet	9	159	33	5	5
Kamut Flakes	1 cup (50g)	6	181	40	7.5	8.5
Muesli	1 cup (85g)	9	290	67	9.4	8.8
Multigrain Bread	1 slice	13	66	12	4	3
Naan Bread	1 piece	11	263	43	8	2.4
Oat Bran Cereal	1 cup (219g)	13	89	26	8	7
Pearl Barley	1 cup (200g)	7	705	156	24	32
Puffed Rice	1 cup (14g)	2	57	13.6	2	1

Puffed Wheat	1 cup (13g)	7	52	12	3	2.7
Quinoa Flakes	1 cup (35g)	19	131	24	5	3.5
Rice Krispies	1 cup (33g)	2	131	30	3	1
Rolled Oats	1 cup (81g)	15	308	56	12	9
Rye Bread	1 slice	9	84	16	3.7	2.9
Rye Crackers	1 oz (28g)	4	109	19	3	5
Shredded Wheat	1 cup (47g)	6	171	41	6	7
Sourdough Bread	1 slice	10	121	24	5	2.3
Spelt Flakes	1 cup (28g)	15	105	23	5	5
Steel Cut Oats	1 cup (156g)	15	171	30	8	6
Sunflower Seeds	1 oz (28g)	10	165	7.5	6.5	4
Wheat Germ	1 oz (28g)	7	102	15	7.5	4.5
Whole Wheat Bread	1 slice	8	70	12	4.5	2.9

Nuts and Seeds

Nuts/Seeds	Portion Size	Oxalate (mg)	Calories	Fat (g)	Protein (g)	Fiber (g)
Black Walnuts	1 oz (28g)	34	184	18	8	3
Brazil Nut Butter	2 tbsp	8	191	19	5	3
Brazil Nuts	1 oz (28g)	4	185	18.8	5	3.1
Cashew Butter	2 tbsp	27	191	15	6	2
Cashews	1 oz (28g)	20	156	12	6	1.9
Chestnuts	1 oz (28g)	5	70	0.6	1.9	2.4
Chia Seed Oil	1 tbsp	3	121	14	1	1
Chia Seeds	1 oz (28g)	3	138	8.6	5.4	11.6
Coconut (Shredded)	1 oz (28g)	2	186	18.1	3	5.6
Flaxseed Oil	1 tbsp	2	121	14	1	1
Flaxseeds	1 oz (28g)	4	151	12	6.1	8.7

Hazelnut Spread	2 tbsp	17	201	11	4	2
Hazelnuts	1 oz (28g)	7	179	17	5.2	3.7
Hemp Seed Butter	2 tbsp	5	167	15	10	2
Hemp Seeds	1 oz (28g)	4	156	13.5	10	2
Lotus Seeds	1 oz (28g)	6	107	0.1	5.7	1
Macadamia Nut Butter	2 tbsp	9	205	22	3	3
Macadamia Nuts	1 oz (28g)	5	205	21.5	3.2	3.4
Peanuts	1 oz (28g)	28	162	14	8.3	3.4
Pecan Butter	2 tbsp	38	191	20	4	2
Pecans	1 oz (28g)	18	197	20.4	3.6	3.7
Pine Nut Oil	1 tbsp	5	121	14	1	1
Pine Nuts	1 oz (28g)	3	192	19	4.9	2
Pistachio Butter	2 tbsp	26	159	12	7	4
Pistachios	1 oz (28g)	14	160	13	7	4
Poppy Seeds	1 oz (28g)	5	127	10	6	7
Pumpkin Seed Oil	1 tbsp	2	121	14	1	1
Pumpkin Seeds	1 oz (28g)	2	159	14	9.5	2.7
Roasted Chestnuts	1 oz (28g)	4	71	0.6	1.9	2.5
Sesame Seed Oil	1 tbsp	82	121	14	1	1
Sesame Seeds	1 oz (28g)	86	161	13.6	6	5.1
Soy Nuts	1 oz (28g)	12	121	6	12	4
Sunflower Seed Butter	2 tbsp	13	167	14	7	3
Sunflower Seeds	1 oz (28g)	5	165	14	6.5	3.4
Tigernuts	1 oz (28g)	15	121	7	3	11
Walnut Oil	1 tbsp	6	121	14	1	1
Walnuts	1 oz (28g)	6	186	18.5	5.3	2.9

Legumes

Legumes	Portion Size	Oxalate (mg)	Calories	Fat (g)	Protein (g)	Fiber (g)
Adzuki Beans	1 cup (230g)	6	295	57	18	18
Alfalfa Sprouts	1 cup (33g)	1	9	1	2	1.6
Anasazi Beans	1 cup (172g)	21	241	44	16	17
Baked Beans (Canned)	1 cup (253g)	11	240	54	13	11
Black Beans	1 cup (172g)	11	228	41	16	16
Black Turtle Beans	1 cup (185g)	21	228	41	16	16
Black-Eyed Peas	1 cup (165g)	21	199	36	14	12
Borlotti Beans	1 cup (182g)	11	241	45	18	16
Cannellini Beans	1 cup (242g)	6	250	45	18	12
Chickpea Flour	1 cup (92g)	21	357	53	21	11
Chickpea Pasta	2 oz (56g)	14	191	32	12	9
Chickpeas (Garbanzo)	1 cup (164g)	15	270	45	16	14
Cowpeas (Black-Eyed Peas)	1 cup (200g)	17	199	36	14	12
Edamame	1 cup (155g)	1	189	16	19	9
Tempeh	1 cup (166g)	11	321	16	32	1
Fava Beans	1 cup (170g)	20	188	33	14	10
Fava Beans (Fresh)	1 cup (170g)	12	188	33	14	10
Garbanzo Beans (Chickpeas)	1 cup (164g)	13	270	45	16	14
Great Northern Beans	1 cup (175g)	7	210	37	16	13
Green Lentils	1 cup (198g)	6	231	40	19	17
Green Mung Beans	1 cup (202g)	7	213	38	15	16
Green Peas (Frozen)	1 cup (160g)	8	118	21	9	8
Hummus	2 tbsp	7	51	5	3	2
Kidney Beans	1 cup (177g)	20	220	40	17	14
Lentil Pasta	2 oz (56g)	11	191	32	14	4
Lentils	1 cup (198g)	15	231	40	19	17
Lima Beans	1 cup (188g)	9	217	39	16	14

Lupini Beans	1 cup (166g)	19	201	16	27	6
Mung Bean Sprouts	1 cup (104g)	4	32	6	4	3
Mung Beans	1 cup (202g)	10	213	38	15	16
Navy Beans	1 cup (182g)	8	256	47	16	20
Navy Beans (Cooked)	1 cup (182g)	3	256	47	16	20
Pea Protein Powder	2 tbsp	2	111	2	26	3
Peanut Butter	2 tbsp	17	189	6	9	3
Peas (Green)	1 cup (145g)	9	118	21	9	8
Pigeon Peas	1 cup (168g)	7	210	39	12	16
Pinto Beans	1 cup (171g)	5	246	45	16	16
Red Kidney Beans	1 cup (177g)	8	226	40	16	12
Red Lentils	1 cup (198g)	12	231	40	19	17
Red Lentils (Cooked)	1 cup (198g)	12	231	40	19	17
Seitan (Wheat Gluten)	3 oz (85g)	1-6	109	5	21	1.5
Soy Milk	1 cup (243g)	6-11	132	15	9	3
Soy Nuts (Roasted)	1 oz (28g)	11-21	121	10	12	4
Soybeans	1 cup (172g)	11-21	299	17	30	11
Soybeans (Cooked)	1 cup (172g)	11-21	299	17	30	11
Split Peas	1 cup (196g)	11-21	232	41	17	17
Tofu (Firm)	1 cup (252g)	11-21	177	12	21	4
White Kidney Beans	1 cup (185g)	6-11	216	40	16	12

Herbs and Spices

Herb/Spice	Portion Size	Oxalate (mg)	Calories	Carbs (g)	Protein (g)	Fiber (g)
Allspice (Ground)	1 tsp	1-3	7	2.5	1.1	1.4
Anise Seed	1 tsp	1-3	8	2	1.3	1.3
Basil (Fresh)	2 tbsp	1-3	2	1	1.1	1.1
Bay Leaves (Dried)	1 leaf	1-3	7	2.4	1.1	1.5
Black Pepper	1 tsp	1-3	6	2.3	1.2	1.5
Caraway Seeds	1 tsp	1-3	8	2	1.3	1.8
Cardamom (Ground)	1 tsp	1-3	7	2.4	1.2	1.6
Cayenne Pepper	1 tsp	1-3	7	2	1.2	1.5
Celery Seed	1 tsp	1-3	9	2	1.4	1.5
Chives (Fresh)	2 tbsp	1-3	2	1.1	1.1	1.1
Cinnamon (Ground)	1 tsp	1-3	7	3	1.1	2.3
Cloves (Ground)	1 tsp	1-3	7	2	1.1	1.5
Coriander (Ground)	1 tsp	1-3	6	2	1.1	1.8
Coriander Leaves	2 tbsp	1-3	2	1.2	1.1	1.2
Cumin (Ground)	1 tsp	1-3	9	2	1.4	1.2
Curry Powder	1 tsp	1-3	7	2	1.2	1.7
Dill (Fresh)	2 tbsp	1-3	2	1.2	1.1	1.1
Fennel Seeds	1 tsp	1-3	8	2	1.3	1.8
Fenugreek Seeds	1 tsp	1-3	13	3.2	1.9	1.9
Garlic Powder	1 tsp	1-3	11	3.3	1.5	1.3
Ginger (Ground)	1 tsp	1-3	7	2.3	1.2	1.2
Horseradish (Fresh)	1 tsp	1-3	3	1.5	1.1	1.2
Kaffir Lime Leaves	1 leaf	1-3	5	2	1.2	1.7
Lemon Balm (Fresh)	2 tbsp	1-3	3	1.4	1.1	1.3
Marjoram (Fresh)	2 tbsp	1-3	2	1.2	1.0	1.1
Mint (Fresh)	2 tbsp	1-3	3	1.5	1.1	1.3
Mustard Seeds	1 tsp	1-3	16	2	2	1.5
Nutmeg (Ground)	1 tsp	1-3	13	2.1	1.1	1.1

Oregano (Dried)	1 tsp	1-3	6	2.2	1.2	1.8
Paprika (Ground)	1 tsp	1-3	7	2.2	1.3	1.8
Parsley (Fresh)	2 tbsp	1-3	3	1.4	1.1	1.1
Rosemary (Fresh)	1 tsp	1-3	2	1.2	1.0	1.1
Saffron	1 tsp	1-3	7	2.3	1.2	1.1
Sage (Fresh)	2 tbsp	1-3	4	1.4	1.1	1.3
Star Anise	1 piece	1-3	24	4	2	1.4
Tarragon (Fresh)	2 tbsp	1-3	3	1.6	1.1	1.1
Thyme (Fresh)	1 tsp	1-3	2	1.2	1.1	1.1
Turmeric (Ground)	1 tsp	1-3	9	2.4	1.2	1.4
Vanilla Bean	1 bean	1-3	21	2	1.1	1.1
White Pepper	1 tsp	1-3	9	3	1.3	1.7

BREAKFAST RECIPES

Oatmeal with Fresh Berries and Almonds

Prep Time: 5 mins

Total Time: 10 mins

Servings: 2

Ingredients

- 1 cup rolled oats
- 2 cups water or low-oxalate milk alternative (e.g., almond milk)
- Pinch of salt
- ½ cup fresh blueberries
- ½ cup sliced strawberries
- ¼ cup sliced almonds
- 1 tablespoon maple syrup or honey (optional)

Directions

1. In a medium saucepan, bring water (or milk alternative) and a pinch of salt to a boil. Add oats and reduce heat to simmer. Cook, stirring occasionally, until the oats are soft and have absorbed most of the liquid, about 5 minutes.
2. Divide the cooked oatmeal into bowls. Top each serving with an equal amount of blueberries, strawberries, and almonds.
3. Drizzle with maple syrup or honey if desired. Serve warm.

Nutrition Facts (per serving)

- Calories: 235
- Fat: 7.5g
- Saturated Fat: 0.9g
- Cholesterol: 0mg
- Sodium: 80mg
- Carbohydrates: 37.2g
- Fiber: 6.7g
- Sugar: 10.3g (natural sugars from fruits; excludes optional maple syrup or honey)
- Protein: 8.1g
- Calcium: 60mg
- Potassium: 240mg

Scrambled Eggs with Spinach and Feta

Prep Time: 5 mins

Total Time: 10 mins

Servings: 2

Ingredients

- 4 large eggs
- 2 tablespoons water
- ½ cup chopped fresh spinach
- ¼ cup crumbled feta cheese
- Salt and pepper to taste
- 1 teaspoon olive oil

Directions

1. In a bowl, whisk together eggs, water, salt, and pepper.
2. Heat olive oil in a non-stick skillet over medium heat. Add the spinach and sauté until just wilted, about 1-2 minutes.
3. Pour the egg mixture over the spinach. Let it sit without stirring for a few seconds, then gently stir and fold the eggs until they form soft curds and are just set, about 2-3 minutes.

4. Sprinkle feta cheese over the eggs, fold gently to mix, and remove from heat.
5. Serve immediately, seasoned with additional salt and pepper if desired.

Nutrition Facts (per serving)
- Calories: 215
- Fat: 15.4g
- Saturated Fat: 6.2g
- Cholesterol: 372mg
- Sodium: 410mg
- Carbohydrates: 2.1g
- Fiber: 0.5g
- Sugar: 1.6g
- Protein: 16.7g
- Calcium: 150mg
- Potassium: 234mg

Avocado Toast with Poached Egg

Prep Time: 10 mins

Total Time: 15 mins

Servings: 2

Ingredients
- 2 slices whole-grain bread (low oxalate option)
- 1 ripe avocado
- Juice of ½ lemon
- Salt and pepper to taste
- 2 eggs
- 1 teaspoon white vinegar

Directions
1. Toast the bread slices to your liking.
2. In a bowl, mash the avocado with lemon juice, salt, and pepper.
3. Spread the mashed avocado evenly on each slice of toasted bread.
4. To poach the eggs, bring a pot of water to a simmer and add vinegar. Crack an egg into a small bowl and gently slide it into the simmering water. Repeat with the second egg. Cook for 3-4 minutes or until the whites are set but yolks remain runny. Use a slotted spoon to remove the eggs from the water.
5. Place a poached egg on top of each avocado toast. Season with additional salt and pepper if desired.
6. Serve immediately.

Nutrition Facts (per serving)
- Calories: 290
- Fat: 19.8g
- Saturated Fat: 4.1g
- Cholesterol: 186mg
- Sodium: 360mg
- Carbohydrates: 19.6g
- Fiber: 7.2g
- Sugar: 3.1g
- Protein: 12.4g
- Calcium: 60mg
- Potassium: 550mg

Cottage Cheese and Pineapple Bowl

Prep Time: 5 mins

Total Time: 5 mins

Servings: 1

Ingredients

- 1 cup low-fat cottage cheese
- ½ cup chopped fresh pineapple
- 1 tablespoon chia seeds

Directions

1. In a serving bowl, place the cottage cheese.
2. Top with chopped pineapple and sprinkle with chia seeds.
3. Serve immediately or chill in the refrigerator for 30 minutes before serving for enhanced flavors.

Nutrition Facts (per serving)

- Calories: 220
- Fat: 5g
- Saturated Fat: 1g
- Cholesterol: 10mg
- Sodium: 500mg
- Carbohydrates: 20g
- Fiber: 3g
- Sugar: 16g
- Protein: 25g
- Calcium: 200mg
- Potassium: 300mg

Quinoa Breakfast Porridge

Prep Time: 5 mins

Total Time: 20 mins

Servings: 2

Ingredients

- 1 cup quinoa, rinsed
- 2 cups water
- 1 apple, peeled and diced
- ½ teaspoon cinnamon
- 1 tablespoon honey or maple syrup
- ¼ cup walnuts, chopped

Directions

1. In a medium saucepan, combine quinoa and water. Bring to a boil, then reduce heat to low, cover, and simmer for 15 minutes, or until quinoa is cooked and water is absorbed.
2. Stir in diced apple, cinnamon, and honey or maple syrup into the cooked quinoa.
3. Divide the porridge between two bowls and top with chopped walnuts.
4. Serve warm.

Nutrition Facts (per serving)

- Calories: 315
- Fat: 9g
- Saturated Fat: 1g
- Cholesterol: 0mg
- Sodium: 13mg
- Carbohydrates: 52g
- Fiber: 6g
- Sugar: 14g

- Protein: 9g
- Calcium: 48mg
- Potassium: 438mg

Baked Avocado Eggs

Prep Time: 5 mins

Total Time: 20 mins

Servings: 2

Ingredients

- 1 large avocado, halved and pitted
- 2 eggs
- Salt and pepper, to taste
- 1 tablespoon chopped chives

Directions

1. Preheat the oven to 425°F (220°C).
2. Scoop out a little more avocado flesh to enlarge the wells.
3. Place avocado halves in a baking dish, ensuring they are stable.
4. Crack an egg into each avocado half. Season with salt and pepper.
5. Bake in the preheated oven for 15 minutes, or until the egg whites are set.
6. Garnish with chopped chives before serving.

Nutrition Facts (per serving)

- Calories: 234
- Fat: 19g
- Saturated Fat: 4g
- Cholesterol: 185mg
- Sodium: 89mg
- Carbohydrates: 9g
- Fiber: 7g
- Sugar: 1g
- Protein: 9g
- Calcium: 35mg
- Potassium: 487mg

Greek Yogurt with Mixed Nuts and Honey

Prep Time: 5 mins

Total Time: 5 mins

Servings: 1

Ingredients

- 1 cup Greek yogurt, unsweetened
- ¼ cup mixed nuts (almonds, walnuts), chopped
- 1 tablespoon honey

Directions

1. In a serving bowl, add the Greek yogurt.
2. Top with chopped mixed nuts.
3. Drizzle honey over the top.
4. Serve immediately or chill for a refreshing breakfast.

Nutrition Facts (per serving)

- Calories: 310
- Fat: 19g
- Saturated Fat: 3g
- Cholesterol: 10mg
- Sodium: 70mg
- Carbohydrates: 18g
- Fiber: 2g
- Sugar: 16g
- Protein: 20g
- Calcium: 180mg
- Potassium: 240mg

Chia Seed Pudding with Kiwi

Prep Time: 15 mins (plus overnight soaking)

Total Time: 15 mins

Servings: 2

Ingredients

- ¼ cup chia seeds
- 1 cup almond milk (unsweetened)
- 1 tablespoon honey or maple syrup (optional)
- ½ teaspoon vanilla extract
- 2 kiwis, peeled and sliced

Directions

1. In a bowl, mix chia seeds, almond milk, honey (or maple syrup), and vanilla extract until well combined.
2. Cover and refrigerate overnight, or at least 6 hours, until it has a pudding-like consistency.
3. Serve the chia pudding in bowls or glasses, topped with sliced kiwi.

Nutrition Facts (per serving)

- Calories: 180
- Fat: 8g
- Saturated Fat: 0.7g
- Cholesterol: 0mg
- Sodium: 80mg
- Carbohydrates: 24g
- Fiber: 10g
- Sugar: 12g (natural sugars from fruit; excludes optional honey/maple syrup)
- Protein: 5g
- Calcium: 350mg
- Potassium: 300mg

Quinoa Breakfast Bowl

Prep Time: 5 mins

Total Time: 20 mins

Servings: 2

Ingredients

- 1 cup quinoa, rinsed
- 2 cups water
- Pinch of salt
- ½ cup almond milk
- 1 apple, diced
- ¼ cup walnuts, chopped
- 2 teaspoons cinnamon

Directions

1. In a saucepan, bring quinoa, water, and a pinch of salt to a boil. Reduce heat to low, cover, and simmer for 15 minutes, or until quinoa is fluffy and water is absorbed.
2. Stir in almond milk, and simmer for an additional 5 minutes.
3. Serve the quinoa in bowls, topped with diced apple, chopped walnuts, and a sprinkle of cinnamon.

Nutrition Facts (per serving)

- Calories: 320
- Fat: 10g
- Saturated Fat: 1g
- Cholesterol: 0mg
- Sodium: 80mg
- Carbohydrates: 50g
- Fiber: 8g
- Sugar: 10g

- Protein: 12g
- Calcium: 100mg
- Potassium: 500mg

Berry Smoothie with Spinach

Prep Time: 5 mins

Total Time: 5 mins

Servings: 2

Ingredients

- 1 cup fresh spinach leaves
- 1 cup mixed berries (strawberries, blueberries, raspberries), fresh or frozen
- 1 banana, sliced
- 1 cup almond milk, unsweetened
- 1 tablespoon flaxseeds, ground

Directions

1. In a blender, combine spinach, mixed berries, banana, almond milk, and ground flaxseeds.
2. Blend on high until smooth and creamy. If the smoothie is too thick, you can add a little more almond milk to reach your desired consistency.
3. Pour the smoothie into glasses and serve immediately.

Nutrition Facts (per serving)

- Calories: 150
- Fat: 3g
- Saturated Fat: 0.3g
- Cholesterol: 0mg
- Sodium: 80mg
- Carbohydrates: 29g
- Fiber: 6g
- Sugar: 16g (natural sugars from fruits)
- Protein: 4g
- Calcium: 200mg
- Potassium: 422mg

MAIN DISH RECIPES

Grilled Chicken with Herb Salad

Prep Time: 15 mins

Total Time: 30 mins

Servings: 4

Ingredients

- 4 boneless, skinless chicken breasts
- 2 tablespoons olive oil
- Salt and pepper to taste
- 1 cup fresh parsley, chopped
- 1 cup fresh basil leaves, chopped
- ½ cup fresh mint leaves, chopped
- 1 tablespoon lemon juice
- 1 teaspoon lemon zest
- 2 tablespoons extra virgin olive oil

Directions

1. Preheat the grill to medium-high heat. Brush chicken breasts with olive oil and season with salt and pepper.
2. Grill chicken for 6-7 minutes on each side or until fully cooked (internal temperature reaches 165°F).
3. In a large bowl, combine parsley, basil, mint, lemon juice, lemon zest, and extra virgin olive oil. Toss gently to mix.
4. Serve grilled chicken topped with the fresh herb salad.

Nutrition Facts (per serving)

- Calories: 290
- Fat: 15g
- Saturated Fat: 2.5g
- Cholesterol: 85mg
- Sodium: 200mg
- Carbohydrates: 2g
- Fiber: 1g
- Sugar: 0g
- Protein: 34g
- Calcium: 60mg
- Potassium: 400mg

Baked Salmon with Asparagus

Prep Time: 10 mins

Total Time: 25 mins

Servings: 4

Ingredients

- 4 salmon fillets (6 ounces each)
- 1 pound asparagus, ends trimmed
- 2 tablespoons olive oil
- Salt and pepper to taste
- 1 lemon, sliced
- 1 tablespoon dill, chopped

Directions

1. Preheat oven to 400°F. Arrange salmon and asparagus on a baking sheet lined with parchment paper.
2. Drizzle olive oil over salmon and asparagus. Season with salt and pepper. Top each salmon fillet with lemon slices.
3. Bake for 15 minutes, or until salmon is cooked through and asparagus is tender.

4. Garnish with chopped dill before serving.

Nutrition Facts (per serving)
- Calories: 345
- Fat: 20g
- Saturated Fat: 3g
- Cholesterol: 95mg
- Sodium: 75mg
- Carbohydrates: 5g
- Fiber: 2g
- Sugar: 2g
- Protein: 35g
- Calcium: 50mg
- Potassium: 900mg

Quinoa Stuffed Bell Peppers

Prep Time: 20 mins

Total Time: 50 mins

Servings: 4

Ingredients
- 4 large bell peppers, halved and seeded
- 1 cup quinoa, cooked
- 1 cup black beans, rinsed and drained
- 1 cup corn kernels, fresh or frozen
- 1 teaspoon cumin
- ½ cup tomato sauce
- Salt and pepper to taste
- ½ cup shredded mozzarella cheese (optional)

Directions
1. Preheat oven to 350°F. Place bell pepper halves in a baking dish, cut-side up.
2. In a bowl, mix quinoa, black beans, corn, cumin, tomato sauce, salt, and pepper.
3. Spoon the mixture into each bell pepper half. Top with shredded cheese if using.
4. Cover with foil and bake for 30 minutes. Uncover and bake for an additional 10 minutes, or until peppers are tender and cheese is melted.

Nutrition Facts (per serving)
- Calories: 280
- Fat: 5g
- Saturated Fat: 2g (if using cheese)
- Cholesterol: 10mg (if using cheese)
- Sodium: 300mg
- Carbohydrates: 45g
- Fiber: 9g
- Sugar: 8g
- Protein: 14g
- Calcium: 150mg
- Potassium: 700mg

Turkey and Vegetable Skillet

Prep Time: 10 mins

Total Time: 30 mins

Servings: 4

Ingredients
- 1 tablespoon olive oil
- 1 pound ground turkey
- 1 onion, diced
- 2 carrots, diced
- 1 zucchini, diced
- 2 cloves garlic, minced
- 1 teaspoon Italian seasoning

- Salt and pepper to taste
- 1 can (14.5 ounces) diced tomatoes, no salt added

Directions

1. Heat olive oil in a large skillet over medium heat. Add ground turkey and cook until browned, breaking it apart with a spoon.
2. Add onion, carrots, zucchini, and garlic. Cook until vegetables are softened, about 5-7 minutes.
3. Stir in Italian seasoning, salt, pepper, and diced tomatoes. Simmer for 10 minutes, or until the mixture thickens slightly.
4. Serve hot, garnished with fresh herbs if desired.

Nutrition Facts (per serving)

- Calories: 250
- Fat: 9g
- Saturated Fat: 2g
- Cholesterol: 65mg
- Sodium: 200mg
- Carbohydrates: 15g
- Fiber: 3g
- Sugar: 7g
- Protein: 28g
- Calcium: 50mg
- Potassium: 650mg

Lentil Soup with Spinach

Prep Time: 15 mins

Total Time: 45 mins

Servings: 4

Ingredients

- 1 tablespoon olive oil
- 1 onion, chopped
- 2 carrots, diced
- 2 stalks celery, diced
- 2 cloves garlic, minced
- 1 cup lentils, rinsed
- 4 cups vegetable broth
- 1 teaspoon ground cumin
- Salt and pepper to taste
- 2 cups fresh spinach leaves
- 1 tablespoon lemon juice

Directions

1. Heat olive oil in a large pot over medium heat. Add onion, carrots, celery, and garlic. Sauté until the vegetables are softened, about 5 minutes.
2. Stir in lentils, vegetable broth, and cumin. Season with salt and pepper. Bring to a boil, then reduce heat and simmer, covered, for 30 minutes, or until lentils are tender.
3. Add spinach to the pot and cook until wilted, about 2 minutes. Stir in lemon juice.
4. Serve hot, with additional lemon wedges on the side if desired.

Nutrition Facts (per serving)
- Calories: 240
- Fat: 4g
- Saturated Fat: 0.5g
- Cholesterol: 0mg
- Sodium: 300mg
- Carbohydrates: 38g
- Fiber: 16g
- Sugar: 5g
- Protein: 14g
- Calcium: 60mg
- Potassium: 710mg

Baked Cod with Roasted Vegetables

Prep Time: 10 mins

Total Time: 30 mins

Servings: 4

Ingredients
- 4 cod fillets (6 ounces each)
- 2 tablespoons olive oil, divided
- Salt and pepper to taste
- 1 zucchini, sliced
- 1 yellow squash, sliced
- 1 red bell pepper, sliced
- 1 tablespoon fresh thyme leaves

Directions
1. Preheat oven to 400°F. Place cod fillets on a baking sheet lined with parchment paper. Brush each fillet with 1 tablespoon olive oil and season with salt and pepper.
2. In a separate bowl, toss zucchini, yellow squash, and red bell pepper with the remaining olive oil and thyme. Season with salt and pepper.
3. Spread the vegetables around the cod on the baking sheet.
4. Bake for 20 minutes, or until the cod is cooked through and vegetables are tender.
5. Serve immediately.

Nutrition Facts (per serving)
- Calories: 220
- Fat: 8g
- Saturated Fat: 1g
- Cholesterol: 60mg
- Sodium: 150mg
- Carbohydrates: 8g
- Fiber: 2g
- Sugar: 4g
- Protein: 29g
- Calcium: 40mg
- Potassium: 700mg

Turkey Meatballs in Tomato Sauce

Prep Time: 20 mins

Total Time: 40 mins

Servings: 4

Ingredients
- 1 pound ground turkey
- 1 egg, beaten
- ¼ cup breadcrumbs
- ¼ cup grated Parmesan cheese
- 1 teaspoon dried oregano
- Salt and pepper to taste
- 2 cups low-sodium tomato sauce
- 1 tablespoon olive oil

Directions

1. In a bowl, mix together ground turkey, egg, breadcrumbs, Parmesan, oregano, salt, and pepper.
2. Form the mixture into 1-inch meatballs.
3. Heat olive oil in a skillet over medium heat. Add meatballs and cook until browned on all sides.
4. Pour tomato sauce over meatballs, cover, and simmer for 20 minutes, or until meatballs are cooked through.
5. Serve hot, garnished with additional Parmesan if desired.

Nutrition Facts (per serving)

- Calories: 290
- Fat: 14g
- Saturated Fat: 3g
- Cholesterol: 120mg
- Sodium: 480mg
- Carbohydrates: 12g
- Fiber: 2g
- Sugar: 4g
- Protein: 31g
- Calcium: 100mg
- Potassium: 500mg

Grilled Vegetable Platter

Prep Time: 15 mins

Total Time: 25 mins

Servings: 4

Ingredients

- 1 eggplant, sliced
- 2 zucchinis, sliced
- 2 red bell peppers, quartered
- 2 tablespoons olive oil
- Salt and pepper to taste
- 1 tablespoon balsamic vinegar
- 1 tablespoon fresh basil, chopped

Directions

1. Preheat grill to medium-high heat.
2. Brush eggplant, zucchinis, and bell peppers with olive oil. Season with salt and pepper.
3. Grill vegetables for 3-4 minutes per side, or until tender and grill marks appear.
4. Arrange grilled vegetables on a platter. Drizzle with balsamic vinegar and sprinkle with fresh basil.
5. Serve warm or at room temperature.

Nutrition Facts (per serving)

- Calories: 120
- Fat: 7g
- Saturated Fat: 1g
- Cholesterol: 0mg
- Sodium: 75mg
- Carbohydrates: 14g
- Fiber: 5g
- Sugar: 9g

- Protein: 3g
- Calcium: 30mg
- Potassium: 520mg

Cauliflower Steak with Herb Sauce

Prep Time: 10 mins

Total Time: 25 mins

Servings: 4

Ingredients

- 2 large heads cauliflower
- 3 tablespoons olive oil, divided
- Salt and pepper to taste
- ½ cup fresh parsley, chopped
- 2 tablespoons fresh chives, chopped
- 1 clove garlic, minced
- Juice of 1 lemon

Directions

1. Preheat oven to 400°F. Slice cauliflower heads into 1-inch thick steaks.
2. Brush cauliflower steaks with 2 tablespoons olive oil and season with salt and pepper. Place on a baking sheet.
3. Roast for 15 minutes, or until tender and golden.
4. In a small bowl, mix together parsley, chives, garlic, lemon juice, and remaining olive oil to create the herb sauce.
5. Serve cauliflower steaks drizzled with herb sauce.

Nutrition Facts (per serving)

- Calories: 180
- Fat: 10g
- Saturated Fat: 1.5g
- Cholesterol: 0mg
- Sodium: 75mg
- Carbohydrates: 20g
- Fiber: 6g
- Sugar: 8g
- Protein: 5g
- Calcium: 60mg
- Potassium: 900mg

Baked Tilapia with Lemon and Dill

Prep Time: 5 mins

Total Time: 20 mins

Servings: 4

Ingredients

- 4 tilapia fillets (6 ounces each)
- 2 tablespoons olive oil
- Salt and pepper to taste
- 1 lemon, thinly sliced
- 2 tablespoons fresh dill, chopped
- 1 garlic clove, minced

Directions

1. Preheat oven to 375°F (190°C). Line a baking sheet with parchment paper.
2. Place tilapia fillets on the prepared baking sheet. Brush each fillet with olive oil and season with salt and pepper.
3. Top each fillet with lemon slices, sprinkle with minced garlic, and garnish with chopped dill.
4. Bake in the preheated oven for 12-15 minutes, or until the fish flakes easily with a fork.

5. Serve immediately, garnished with additional fresh dill if desired.

Nutrition Facts (per serving)
- Calories: 210
- Fat: 10g
- Saturated Fat: 1.5g
- Cholesterol: 85mg
- Sodium: 100mg
- Carbohydrates: 2g
- Fiber: 0.5g
- Sugar: 0g
- Protein: 30g
- Calcium: 20mg
- Potassium: 450mg

SNACKS RECIPES

Cucumber and Hummus Bites

Prep Time: 10 mins

Total Time: 10 mins

Servings: 4

Ingredients

- 2 large cucumbers, sliced into rounds
- 1 cup hummus
- Paprika for garnish
- Fresh parsley, chopped for garnish

Directions

1. Lay cucumber rounds on a serving platter.
2. Spoon a dollop of hummus onto each cucumber round.
3. Sprinkle a light dusting of paprika over the hummus and garnish with chopped parsley.
4. Serve immediately or chill until serving.

Nutrition Facts (per serving)

- Calories: 105
- Fat: 5.5g
- Saturated Fat: 0.9g
- Cholesterol: 0mg
- Sodium: 198mg
- Carbohydrates: 12.4g
- Fiber: 5.1g
- Sugar: 2.1g
- Protein: 4.9g
- Calcium: 49mg
- Potassium: 310mg

Apple Slices with Almond Butter

Prep Time: 5 mins

Total Time: 5 mins

Servings: 4

Ingredients

- 2 large apples, cored and sliced
- ¼ cup almond butter

Directions

1. Arrange apple slices on a plate.
2. Serve with almond butter for dipping.
3. Enjoy as a crunchy and creamy snack.

Nutrition Facts (per serving)

- Calories: 150
- Fat: 8.2g
- Saturated Fat: 1.5g
- Cholesterol: 0mg
- Sodium: 3mg
- Carbohydrates: 18.5g
- Fiber: 4.2g
- Sugar: 13.2g
- Protein: 3.5g
- Calcium: 76mg
- Potassium: 239mg

Greek Yogurt with Honey and Walnuts

Prep Time: 5 mins

Total Time: 5 mins

Servings: 4

Ingredients

- 2 cups Greek yogurt, plain
- 4 tablespoons honey
- ½ cup walnuts, chopped

Directions

1. Divide Greek yogurt into serving bowls.
2. Drizzle each serving with 1 tablespoon of honey.
3. Sprinkle chopped walnuts on top.
4. Serve immediately for a creamy and crunchy snack.

Nutrition Facts (per serving)

- Calories: 245
- Fat: 12g
- Saturated Fat: 2g
- Cholesterol: 10mg
- Sodium: 36mg
- Carbohydrates: 24g
- Fiber: 1.5g
- Sugar: 21g
- Protein: 12g
- Calcium: 150mg
- Potassium: 200mg

Carrot Sticks with Avocado Dip

Prep Time: 15 mins

Total Time: 15 mins

Servings: 4

Ingredients

- 4 large carrots, peeled and cut into sticks
- 1 ripe avocado
- Juice of 1 lime
- Salt and pepper to taste

Directions

1. Mash the avocado in a bowl and mix with lime juice, salt, and pepper to create a smooth dip.
2. Serve carrot sticks alongside the avocado dip.
3. Enjoy a refreshing and healthy snack.

Nutrition Facts (per serving)

- Calories: 114
- Fat: 7.4g
- Saturated Fat: 1.1g
- Cholesterol: 0mg
- Sodium: 89mg
- Carbohydrates: 12.3g
- Fiber: 6.2g
- Sugar: 5.1g
- Protein: 2.1g
- Calcium: 33mg
- Potassium: 487mg

Baked Kale Chips

Prep Time: 10 mins

Total Time: 25 mins

Servings: 4

Ingredients

- 1 bunch kale, washed, dried, and torn into bite-sized pieces
- 1 tablespoon olive oil
- Salt to taste

Directions

1. Preheat oven to 300°F (150°C). Line a baking sheet with parchment paper.
2. In a large bowl, toss kale pieces with olive oil and salt until evenly coated.
3. Spread kale in a single layer on the prepared baking sheet.
4. Bake for 15 minutes, or until crisp, turning halfway through.
5. Serve immediately as a crunchy, low-oxalate snack.

Nutrition Facts (per serving)

- Calories: 58
- Fat: 3.5g
- Saturated Fat: 0.5g
- Cholesterol: 0mg
- Sodium: 50mg
- Carbohydrates: 6.4g
- Fiber: 1.2g
- Sugar: 1.5g
- Protein: 2.2g
- Calcium: 53mg
- Potassium: 212mg

Roasted Chickpeas

Prep Time: 10 mins

Total Time: 40 mins

Servings: 4

Ingredients

- 1 can (15 ounces) chickpeas, drained, rinsed, and patted dry
- 1 tablespoon olive oil
- ½ teaspoon paprika
- Salt to taste

Directions

1. Preheat oven to 400°F (200°C). Line a baking sheet with parchment paper.
2. Toss chickpeas with olive oil, paprika, and salt in a bowl until evenly coated.
3. Spread chickpeas in a single layer on the prepared baking sheet.
4. Roast for 30 minutes, stirring halfway through, until crispy and golden.
5. Let cool before serving as a crunchy, protein-rich snack.

Nutrition Facts (per serving)

- Calories: 134
- Fat: 5g
- Saturated Fat: 0.6g
- Cholesterol: 0mg
- Sodium: 300mg
- Carbohydrates: 18g
- Fiber: 5g
- Sugar: 3g
- Protein: 6g

- Calcium: 49mg
- Potassium: 210mg

Zucchini Chips

Prep Time: 15 mins

Total Time: 2 hours

Servings: 4

Ingredients
- 2 large zucchinis, thinly sliced
- 1 tablespoon olive oil
- Salt to taste

Directions
1. Preheat oven to 225°F (105°C). Line a baking sheet with parchment paper.
2. Toss zucchini slices with olive oil and salt until evenly coated.
3. Arrange zucchini slices in a single layer on the baking sheet.
4. Bake for 1½ to 2 hours, flipping the slices halfway through, until crispy.
5. Cool before serving as a light and healthy snack.

Nutrition Facts (per serving)
- Calories: 60
- Fat: 3.5g
- Saturated Fat: 0.5g
- Cholesterol: 0mg
- Sodium: 75mg
- Carbohydrates: 6g
- Fiber: 2g
- Sugar: 4g
- Protein: 2g
- Calcium: 22mg

- Potassium: 512mg

Peanut Butter Banana Bites

Prep Time: 15 mins

Total Time: 1 hour 15 mins (includes freezing)

Servings: 4

Ingredients
- 2 bananas, sliced
- ¼ cup natural peanut butter
- 1 tablespoon coconut oil, melted

Directions
1. Line a baking sheet with parchment paper.
2. Sandwich a small amount of peanut butter between two banana slices. Repeat with remaining banana slices and peanut butter.
3. Freeze banana bites for 1 hour.
4. Drizzle with melted coconut oil before serving.
5. Enjoy as a frozen treat or snack.

Nutrition Facts (per serving)
- Calories: 188
- Fat: 11g
- Saturated Fat: 4g
- Cholesterol: 0mg
- Sodium: 76mg
- Carbohydrates: 21g
- Fiber: 3g
- Sugar: 11g
- Protein: 4g
- Calcium: 10mg
- Potassium: 322mg

Cucumber Roll-Ups with Hummus

Prep Time: 20 mins

Total Time: 20 mins

Servings: 4

Ingredients

- 1 large cucumber, thinly sliced lengthwise
- 1 cup hummus
- ¼ cup shredded carrots
- ¼ cup thinly sliced red bell pepper

Directions

1. Spread a thin layer of hummus over each cucumber slice.
2. Place a small amount of shredded carrots and red bell pepper at one end of each cucumber slice.
3. Carefully roll up the cucumber slices.
4. Serve immediately as a fresh and crunchy snack.

Nutrition Facts (per serving)

- Calories: 105
- Fat: 5.5g
- Saturated Fat: 0.8g
- Cholesterol: 0mg
- Sodium: 198mg
- Carbohydrates: 12g
- Fiber: 3.5g
- Sugar: 2g
- Protein: 3.5g
- Calcium: 30mg
- Potassium: 220mg

Avocado Toast with Cherry Tomatoes

Prep Time: 5 mins

Total Time: 5 mins

Servings: 4

Ingredients

- 4 slices whole-grain bread, toasted
- 2 ripe avocados, mashed
- 1 cup cherry tomatoes, halved
- Salt and pepper to taste
- 1 teaspoon lemon juice

Directions

1. Spread mashed avocado evenly on each slice of toasted bread.
2. Top with cherry tomato halves.
3. Season with salt, pepper, and a drizzle of lemon juice.
4. Serve immediately as a nutritious and satisfying snack.

Nutrition Facts (per serving)

- Calories: 250
- Fat: 15g
- Saturated Fat: 2.2g
- Cholesterol: 0mg
- Sodium: 200mg
- Carbohydrates: 27g
- Fiber: 9g
- Sugar: 5g
- Protein: 6g
- Calcium: 40mg
- Potassium: 690mg

VEGETABLES AND SALAD

Mixed Greens with Apple and Walnuts

Prep Time: 10 mins

Total Time: 10 mins

Servings: 4

Ingredients

- 6 cups mixed greens (spinach, arugula, and lettuce)
- 1 large apple, cored and thinly sliced
- ½ cup walnuts, chopped
- ¼ cup crumbled feta cheese
- 2 tablespoons olive oil
- 1 tablespoon balsamic vinegar
- Salt and pepper to taste

Directions

1. In a large salad bowl, combine mixed greens, apple slices, and chopped walnuts.
2. Sprinkle crumbled feta cheese over the salad.
3. In a small bowl, whisk together olive oil and balsamic vinegar with a pinch of salt and pepper to create the dressing.
4. Drizzle the dressing over the salad and toss gently to coat.
5. Serve immediately, offering a refreshing blend of sweet and savory flavors.

Nutrition Facts (per serving)

- Calories: 220
- Fat: 18g
- Saturated Fat: 3g
- Cholesterol: 8mg
- Sodium: 180mg
- Carbohydrates: 12g
- Fiber: 3g
- Sugar: 7g
- Protein: 5g
- Calcium: 90mg
- Potassium: 300mg

Cucumber Tomato Salad

Prep Time: 15 mins

Total Time: 15 mins

Servings: 4

Ingredients

- 2 large cucumbers, diced
- 3 medium tomatoes, diced
- ¼ cup red onion, thinly sliced
- ¼ cup fresh parsley, chopped
- 2 tablespoons olive oil
- 1 tablespoon lemon juice
- Salt and pepper to taste

Directions

1. In a large bowl, combine cucumbers, tomatoes, red onion, and parsley.
2. In a small bowl, whisk together olive oil, lemon juice, salt, and pepper to create the dressing.
3. Pour the dressing over the salad and toss to combine.

4. Chill for about 10 minutes before serving to allow flavors to meld.

Nutrition Facts (per serving)
- Calories: 110
- Fat: 7g
- Saturated Fat: 1g
- Cholesterol: 0mg
- Sodium: 10mg
- Carbohydrates: 11g
- Fiber: 3g
- Sugar: 6g
- Protein: 2g
- Calcium: 30mg
- Potassium: 420mg

Roasted Beet and Goat Cheese Salad

Prep Time: 10 mins (plus roasting time)

Total Time: 1 hr

Servings: 4

Ingredients
- 4 medium beets, roasted, peeled, and sliced
- 4 cups mixed salad greens
- ½ cup goat cheese, crumbled
- ¼ cup walnuts, toasted and chopped
- 2 tablespoons olive oil
- 1 tablespoon red wine vinegar
- Salt and pepper to taste

Directions
1. Preheat the oven to 400°F. Wrap beets in foil and roast until tender, about 45-50 minutes. Let cool, then peel and slice.
2. Arrange mixed salad greens on a platter. Top with sliced beets, crumbled goat cheese, and toasted walnuts.
3. In a small bowl, whisk together olive oil, red wine vinegar, salt, and pepper to create the dressing.
4. Drizzle the dressing over the salad just before serving.

Nutrition Facts (per serving)
- Calories: 250
- Fat: 18g
- Saturated Fat: 6g
- Cholesterol: 13mg
- Sodium: 240mg
- Carbohydrates: 14g
- Fiber: 4g
- Sugar: 9g
- Protein: 9g
- Calcium: 70mg
- Potassium: 500mg

Carrot Slaw with Cranberries

Prep Time: 15 mins

Total Time: 15 mins

Servings: 4

Ingredients
- 4 cups shredded carrots
- ½ cup dried cranberries
- ¼ cup slivered almonds
- 3 tablespoons olive oil
- 2 tablespoons apple cider vinegar
- 1 tablespoon honey
- Salt and pepper to taste

Directions
1. In a large bowl, combine shredded carrots, dried cranberries, and slivered almonds.
2. In a small bowl, whisk together olive oil, apple cider vinegar, honey, salt, and pepper to create the dressing.
3. Pour the dressing over the carrot mixture and toss to coat evenly.
4. Serve immediately or chill in the refrigerator for 1 hour before serving to enhance the flavors.

Nutrition Facts (per serving)
- Calories: 210
- Fat: 12g
- Saturated Fat: 1.5g
- Cholesterol: 0mg
- Sodium: 85mg
- Carbohydrates: 27g
- Fiber: 5g
- Sugar: 19g
- Protein: 3g
- Calcium: 60mg
- Potassium: 360mg

Spinach and Strawberry Salad

Prep Time: 10 mins
Total Time: 10 mins
Servings: 4

Ingredients
- 6 cups fresh spinach leaves
- 1 cup strawberries, sliced
- ½ cup walnuts, toasted
- ¼ cup feta cheese, crumbled
- 2 tablespoons balsamic vinegar
- 1 tablespoon olive oil
- 1 teaspoon honey
- Salt and pepper to taste

Directions
1. In a large salad bowl, combine spinach, sliced strawberries, toasted walnuts, and crumbled feta cheese.
2. In a small bowl, whisk together balsamic vinegar, olive oil, honey, salt, and pepper to create the dressing.
3. Drizzle the dressing over the salad and toss gently to combine.
4. Serve immediately, offering a delightful blend of sweet and savory flavors.

Nutrition Facts (per serving)
- Calories: 210
- Fat: 16g
- Saturated Fat: 3g
- Cholesterol: 8mg
- Sodium: 180mg
- Carbohydrates: 14g
- Fiber: 3g

- Sugar: 9g
- Protein: 5g
- Calcium: 90mg
- Potassium: 320mg

Avocado and Tomato Salad

Prep Time: 10 mins

Total Time: 10 mins

Servings: 4

Ingredients

- 2 ripe avocados, diced
- 2 large tomatoes, diced
- ¼ cup red onion, finely chopped
- 2 tablespoons cilantro, chopped
- Juice of 1 lime
- Salt and pepper to taste

Directions

1. In a salad bowl, combine diced avocados, tomatoes, red onion, and cilantro.
2. Squeeze lime juice over the salad and season with salt and pepper.
3. Toss gently to mix. Serve immediately to enjoy the fresh flavors.

Nutrition Facts (per serving)

- Calories: 170
- Fat: 14g
- Saturated Fat: 2g
- Cholesterol: 0mg
- Sodium: 10mg
- Carbohydrates: 12g
- Fiber: 7g
- Sugar: 3g
- Protein: 2g
- Calcium: 20mg
- Potassium: 490mg

Broccoli and Cauliflower Salad

Prep Time: 15 mins

Total Time: 15 mins

Servings: 4

Ingredients

- 2 cups broccoli florets
- 2 cups cauliflower florets
- ¼ cup sunflower seeds
- ¼ cup raisins
- ¼ cup low-fat mayonnaise
- 2 tablespoons white vinegar
- 1 tablespoon sugar
- Salt and pepper to taste

Directions

1. In a large bowl, combine broccoli, cauliflower, sunflower seeds, and raisins.
2. In a small bowl, whisk together mayonnaise, vinegar, sugar, salt, and pepper to create the dressing.
3. Pour the dressing over the vegetable mixture and toss to coat evenly.
4. Chill in the refrigerator for at least 1 hour before serving to allow flavors to meld.

Nutrition Facts (per serving)

- Calories: 180
- Fat: 9g
- Saturated Fat: 1g
- Cholesterol: 5mg
- Sodium: 200mg
- Carbohydrates: 24g

- Fiber: 3g
- Sugar: 15g
- Protein: 3g
- Calcium: 40mg
- Potassium: 350mg

Cucumber Dill Salad

Prep Time: 10 mins

Total Time: 1 hr 10 mins (includes chilling)

Servings: 4

Ingredients

- 3 large cucumbers, thinly sliced
- ¼ cup red onion, thinly sliced
- ½ cup plain yogurt
- 2 tablespoons fresh dill, chopped
- 1 tablespoon lemon juice
- Salt and pepper to taste

Directions

1. In a salad bowl, combine cucumbers and red onion.
2. In a small bowl, mix yogurt, dill, lemon juice, salt, and pepper to create the dressing.
3. Pour the dressing over the cucumbers and onions, tossing to coat.
4. Refrigerate for 1 hour before serving to enhance the flavors.

Nutrition Facts (per serving)

- Calories: 70
- Fat: 1g
- Saturated Fat: 0.5g
- Cholesterol: 3mg
- Sodium: 30mg
- Carbohydrates: 13g
- Fiber: 2g
- Sugar: 6g
- Protein: 3g
- Calcium: 80mg
- Potassium: 440mg

Mixed Bean Salad

Prep Time: 15 mins

Total Time: 15 mins

Servings: 4

Ingredients

- 1 can (15 ounces) low-sodium black beans, rinsed and drained
- 1 can (15 ounces) low-sodium chickpeas, rinsed and drained
- 1 red bell pepper, diced
- ¼ cup fresh parsley, chopped
- 2 tablespoons olive oil
- 1 tablespoon red wine vinegar
- 1 garlic clove, minced
- Salt and pepper to taste

Directions

1. In a salad bowl, combine black beans, chickpeas, red bell pepper, and parsley.
2. In a small bowl, whisk together olive oil, red wine vinegar, minced garlic, salt, and pepper to create the dressing.
3. Pour the dressing over the bean mixture and toss to combine.
4. Serve immediately or chill in the refrigerator to allow flavors to meld.

Nutrition Facts (per serving)
- Calories: 220
- Fat: 7g
- Saturated Fat: 1g
- Cholesterol: 0mg
- Sodium: 200mg
- Carbohydrates: 30g
- Fiber: 9g
- Sugar: 5g
- Protein: 10g
- Calcium: 60mg
- Potassium: 460mg

Shaved Brussels Sprout Salad

Prep Time: 20 mins

Total Time: 20 mins

Servings: 4

Ingredients
- 4 cups Brussels sprouts, trimmed and thinly sliced
- 1 apple, cored and thinly sliced
- 1/4 cup dried cranberries
- 1/4 cup chopped walnuts
- 1/4 cup grated Parmesan cheese
- 2 tablespoons olive oil
- 1 tablespoon apple cider vinegar
- 1 teaspoon Dijon mustard
- Salt and pepper to taste

Directions
1. In a large bowl, combine the shaved Brussels sprouts, sliced apple, dried cranberries, chopped walnuts, and grated Parmesan cheese.
2. In a small bowl, whisk together the olive oil, apple cider vinegar, Dijon mustard, salt, and pepper to create the dressing.
3. Pour the dressing over the salad ingredients in the large bowl. Toss well to ensure all the ingredients are evenly coated with the dressing.
4. Let the salad sit for about 10 minutes before serving to allow the flavors to meld together.
5. Serve as a fresh, crunchy side dish or a light main course.

Nutrition Facts (per serving)
- Calories: 210
- Fat: 14g
- Saturated Fat: 3g
- Cholesterol: 5mg
- Sodium: 170mg
- Carbohydrates: 19g
- Fiber: 4g
- Sugar: 10g
- Protein: 6g
- Calcium: 100mg
- Potassium: 450mg

SOUP AND STEW

Chicken and Rice Soup

Prep Time: 10 mins

Total Time: 40 mins

Servings: 4

Ingredients

- 1 tablespoon olive oil
- 1 onion, chopped
- 2 carrots, peeled and diced
- 2 celery stalks, diced
- 2 garlic cloves, minced
- 1 pound chicken breast, cubed
- 6 cups low-sodium chicken broth
- 1 cup brown rice, rinsed
- Salt and pepper to taste
- 2 tablespoons fresh parsley, chopped

Directions

1. Heat olive oil in a large pot over medium heat. Add onion, carrots, celery, and garlic. Sauté until vegetables are softened, about 5 minutes.
2. Add cubed chicken to the pot and cook until no longer pink, about 5-7 minutes.
3. Pour in chicken broth and bring to a boil. Add brown rice, reduce heat to low, cover, and simmer for 25 minutes, or until rice is tender.
4. Season with salt and pepper to taste. Stir in fresh parsley just before serving.
5. Serve hot, offering a comforting and nutritious meal.

Nutrition Facts (per serving)
- Calories: 290
- Fat: 6g
- Saturated Fat: 1g
- Cholesterol: 65mg
- Sodium: 150mg
- Carbohydrates: 30g
- Fiber: 3g
- Sugar: 3g
- Protein: 28g
- Calcium: 40mg
- Potassium: 600mg

Tomato Basil Soup

Prep Time: 5 mins

Total Time: 25 mins

Servings: 4

Ingredients

- 1 tablespoon olive oil
- 1 onion, chopped
- 2 garlic cloves, minced
- 1 can (28 ounces) no-salt-added diced tomatoes
- 2 cups vegetable broth
- 1/4 cup fresh basil, chopped
- Salt and pepper to taste
- 1/4 cup low-fat milk (optional)

Directions

1. In a large pot, heat olive oil over medium heat. Add onion and garlic, sautéing until softened, about 5 minutes.
2. Add diced tomatoes (with juice) and vegetable broth. Bring to a simmer and cook for 15 minutes.
3. Stir in chopped basil, and season with salt and pepper.
4. Use an immersion blender to puree the soup until smooth. Stir in milk for a creamier texture if desired.
5. Serve hot, garnished with additional basil leaves.

Nutrition Facts (per serving)
- Calories: 90
- Fat: 3.5g
- Saturated Fat: 0.5g
- Cholesterol: 1mg
- Sodium: 200mg
- Carbohydrates: 13g
- Fiber: 3g
- Sugar: 7g
- Protein: 3g
- Calcium: 60mg
- Potassium: 430mg

Lentil Vegetable Stew

Prep Time: 15 mins
Total Time: 45 mins
Servings: 4

Ingredients
- 1 tablespoon olive oil
- 1 onion, chopped
- 2 carrots, peeled and diced
- 2 celery stalks, diced
- 2 garlic cloves, minced
- 1 cup lentils, rinsed
- 4 cups low-sodium vegetable broth
- 1 can (14 ounces) no-salt-added diced tomatoes
- 1 teaspoon thyme
- Salt and pepper to taste
- 2 cups spinach leaves

Directions

1. Heat olive oil in a large pot over medium heat. Add onion, carrots, celery, and garlic. Sauté until vegetables are softened, about 5 minutes.
2. Add lentils, vegetable broth, diced tomatoes (with juice), and thyme. Season with salt and pepper.
3. Bring to a boil, then reduce heat to low, cover, and simmer for 30 minutes, or until lentils are tender.
4. Stir in spinach and cook until wilted, about 2 minutes.
5. Serve hot, offering a hearty and healthy stew.

Nutrition Facts (per serving)
- Calories: 250
- Fat: 4g
- Saturated Fat: 0.5g
- Cholesterol: 0mg
- Sodium: 200mg

- Carbohydrates: 40g
- Fiber: 15g
- Sugar: 7g
- Protein: 14g
- Calcium: 60mg
- Potassium: 800mg

Butternut Squash Soup

Prep Time: 20 mins

Total Time: 45 mins

Servings: 4

Ingredients

- 1 tablespoon olive oil
- 1 onion, chopped
- 1 butternut squash, peeled, seeded, and cubed
- 4 cups low-sodium vegetable broth
- Salt and pepper to taste
- 1/2 teaspoon nutmeg
- 1/4 cup low-fat coconut milk

Directions

1. In a large pot, heat olive oil over medium heat. Add onion and sauté until translucent, about 5 minutes.
2. Add cubed butternut squash and vegetable broth. Season with salt, pepper, and nutmeg.
3. Bring to a boil, then reduce heat to low, cover, and simmer for 30 minutes, or until squash is tender.
4. Use an immersion blender to puree the soup until smooth. Stir in coconut milk for a creamy texture.
5. Serve hot, garnished with a sprinkle of nutmeg or fresh herbs.

Nutrition Facts (per serving)

- Calories: 180
- Fat: 5g
- Saturated Fat: 1g
- Cholesterol: 0mg
- Sodium: 150mg
- Carbohydrates: 33g
- Fiber: 5g
- Sugar: 8g
- Protein: 3g
- Calcium: 80mg
- Potassium: 790mg

Carrot Ginger Soup

Prep Time: 10 mins

Total Time: 30 mins

Servings: 4

Ingredients

- 2 tablespoons olive oil
- 1 onion, diced
- 2 pounds carrots, peeled and chopped
- 2 tablespoons grated fresh ginger
- 4 cups low-sodium vegetable broth
- Salt and pepper to taste
- 1/4 cup coconut milk for garnish (optional)

Directions

1. In a large pot, heat olive oil over medium heat. Add onion and sauté until translucent, about 5 minutes.

2. Add carrots and ginger, cooking for another 5 minutes until carrots start to soften.
3. Pour in vegetable broth, season with salt and pepper, and bring to a boil. Reduce heat and simmer for 20 minutes, or until carrots are very tender.
4. Use an immersion blender to puree the soup until smooth.
5. Serve hot, drizzled with coconut milk if desired.

Nutrition Facts (per serving)
- Calories: 190
- Fat: 7g
- Saturated Fat: 1g
- Cholesterol: 0mg
- Sodium: 300mg
- Carbohydrates: 29g
- Fiber: 8g
- Sugar: 13g
- Protein: 3g
- Calcium: 80mg
- Potassium: 790mg

Zucchini Basil Soup

Prep Time: 5 mins

Total Time: 20 mins

Servings: 4

Ingredients
- 1 tablespoon olive oil
- 1 small onion, chopped
- 3 zucchinis, sliced
- 4 cups low-sodium vegetable broth
- 1/4 cup fresh basil leaves
- Salt and pepper to taste

Directions
1. In a large pot, heat olive oil over medium heat. Add onion and sauté until soft, about 5 minutes.
2. Add zucchini and cook for another 5 minutes.
3. Pour in vegetable broth and bring to a simmer. Cook until zucchini is tender, about 10 minutes.
4. Stir in fresh basil and use an immersion blender to puree the soup until smooth.
5. Season with salt and pepper to taste. Serve hot.

Nutrition Facts (per serving)
- Calories: 80
- Fat: 4g
- Saturated Fat: 0.5g
- Cholesterol: 0mg
- Sodium: 200mg
- Carbohydrates: 10g
- Fiber: 3g
- Sugar: 6g
- Protein: 3g
- Calcium: 30mg
- Potassium: 510mg

Creamy Mushroom Soup

Prep Time: 10 mins

Total Time: 30 mins

Servings: 4

Ingredients

- 2 tablespoons olive oil
- 1 onion, diced
- 2 garlic cloves, minced
- 1 pound mushrooms, sliced
- 4 cups low-sodium vegetable broth
- 1 teaspoon thyme
- Salt and pepper to taste
- 1/4 cup low-fat sour cream

Directions

1. In a large pot, heat olive oil over medium heat. Add onion and garlic, sautéing until softened.
2. Add mushrooms and thyme, cooking until mushrooms are browned and their liquid has evaporated.
3. Pour in vegetable broth and bring to a simmer. Cook for 15 minutes.
4. Stir in sour cream and use an immersion blender to blend the soup until smooth.
5. Season with salt and pepper. Serve hot.

Nutrition Facts (per serving)

- Calories: 150
- Fat: 9g
- Saturated Fat: 2g
- Cholesterol: 10mg
- Sodium: 200mg
- Carbohydrates: 13g
- Fiber: 2g
- Sugar: 6g
- Protein: 6g
- Calcium: 50mg
- Potassium: 600mg

Sweet Potato and Lentil Stew

Prep Time: 15 mins

Total Time: 45 mins

Servings: 4

Ingredients

- 1 tablespoon olive oil
- 1 onion, chopped
- 2 garlic cloves, minced
- 1 large sweet potato, peeled and cubed
- 1 cup lentils, rinsed
- 4 cups low-sodium vegetable broth
- 1 teaspoon cumin
- Salt and pepper to taste
- 2 cups spinach leaves

Directions

1. In a large pot, heat olive oil over medium heat. Add onion and garlic, and sauté until soft.
2. Add sweet potato, lentils, vegetable broth, and cumin. Season with salt and pepper.
3. Bring to a boil, then reduce heat and simmer, covered, for 30 minutes or until lentils and sweet potatoes are tender.
4. Stir in spinach until wilted.
5. Serve hot, offering a hearty and nutritious meal.

Nutrition Facts (per serving)
- Calories: 240
- Fat: 4g
- Saturated Fat: 0.5g
- Cholesterol: 0mg
- Sodium: 300mg
- Carbohydrates: 40g
- Fiber: 15g
- Sugar: 7g
- Protein: 14g
- Calcium: 60mg
- Potassium: 800mg

Creamy Cauliflower Soup

Prep Time: 10 mins

Total Time: 35 mins

Servings: 4

Ingredients
- 1 tablespoon olive oil
- 1 medium onion, diced
- 2 cloves garlic, minced
- 1 head cauliflower, chopped into florets
- 4 cups low-sodium vegetable broth
- ½ teaspoon dried thyme
- Salt and pepper to taste
- ¼ cup low-fat cream or milk alternative

Directions
1. In a large pot, heat olive oil over medium heat. Add onion and garlic, sautéing until translucent, about 5 minutes.
2. Add cauliflower florets, vegetable broth, thyme, salt, and pepper. Bring to a boil, then reduce heat and simmer for 25 minutes, or until cauliflower is very tender.
3. Use an immersion blender to puree the soup until smooth. Stir in the cream or milk alternative and heat through.
4. Adjust seasoning as needed and serve hot, garnished with a sprinkle of fresh herbs or a drizzle of olive oil.

Nutrition Facts (per serving)
- Calories: 120
- Fat: 4g
- Saturated Fat: 1g
- Cholesterol: 5mg
- Sodium: 200mg
- Carbohydrates: 17g
- Fiber: 5g
- Sugar: 8g
- Protein: 5g
- Calcium: 60mg
- Potassium: 500mg

Chicken Vegetable Soup

Prep Time: 15 mins

Total Time: 45 mins

Servings: 4

Ingredients
- 1 tablespoon olive oil
- 1 small onion, chopped
- 2 medium carrots, peeled and diced
- 2 stalks celery, diced
- 2 cloves garlic, minced

- 1 pound boneless, skinless chicken breasts, cut into bite-sized pieces
- 6 cups low-sodium chicken broth
- 1 teaspoon dried thyme
- 1 bay leaf
- Salt and pepper to taste
- 1 cup green beans, trimmed and cut into 1-inch pieces
- 2 tablespoons fresh parsley, chopped

Directions

1. In a large pot, heat olive oil over medium heat. Add onion, carrots, celery, and garlic. Cook, stirring occasionally, until the vegetables are softened, about 5 minutes.
2. Add chicken pieces to the pot and cook until no longer pink on the outside, about 5 minutes.
3. Pour in chicken broth and add thyme and bay leaf. Season with salt and pepper. Bring to a boil, then reduce heat and simmer for 20 minutes.
4. Add green beans to the pot and simmer for an additional 10 minutes, or until the beans are tender and the chicken is fully cooked.
5. Remove the bay leaf, stir in fresh parsley, and adjust seasoning as needed.
6. Serve hot, enjoying a classic and comforting soup.

Nutrition Facts (per serving)

- Calories: 220
- Fat: 6g
- Saturated Fat: 1g
- Cholesterol: 55mg
- Sodium: 300mg
- Carbohydrates: 14g
- Fiber: 3g
- Sugar: 5g
- Protein: 29g
- Calcium: 50mg
- Potassium: 700mg

DESSERT RECIPES

Baked Apples with Cinnamon

Prep Time: 10 mins

Total Time: 50 mins

Servings: 4

Ingredients

- 4 large apples, cored
- 4 teaspoons unsalted butter
- 2 teaspoons cinnamon
- 4 teaspoons honey
- ½ cup water

Directions

1. Preheat oven to 350°F (175°C). Place the cored apples in a baking dish.
2. Place 1 teaspoon of butter in the center of each apple. Sprinkle evenly with cinnamon and drizzle each with 1 teaspoon of honey.
3. Pour water into the bottom of the baking dish to help keep the apples moist while baking.
4. Bake in the preheated oven for 40 minutes, or until apples are soft and tender.
5. Serve warm, spooning the juices from the baking dish over the apples.

Nutrition Facts (per serving)

- Calories: 150
- Fat: 4g
- Saturated Fat: 2.5g
- Cholesterol: 10mg
- Sodium: 5mg
- Carbohydrate: 31g
- Fiber: 5g
- Sugar: 24g
- Protein: 0g
- Calcium: 20mg
- Potassium: 195mg

Vanilla Rice Pudding

Prep Time: 5 mins

Total Time: 35 mins

Servings: 4

Ingredients

- 1 cup cooked white rice
- 2 cups low-fat milk
- ¼ cup sugar
- 1 teaspoon vanilla extract
- Pinch of salt
- Ground cinnamon for garnish

Directions

1. In a saucepan, combine cooked rice, milk, sugar, and a pinch of salt. Cook over medium heat, stirring frequently until thick and creamy, about 30 minutes.
2. Remove from heat and stir in vanilla extract.
3. Divide the pudding into serving dishes and refrigerate until set, about 1 hour.
4. Sprinkle with ground cinnamon before serving.

Nutrition Facts (per serving)

- Calories: 180

- Fat: 2g
- Saturated Fat: 1g
- Cholesterol: 5mg
- Sodium: 60mg
- Carbohydrate: 36g
- Fiber: 0g
- Sugar: 22g
- Protein: 5g
- Calcium: 150mg
- Potassium: 210mg

Peach Yogurt Parfait

Prep Time: 10 mins

Total Time: 10 mins

Servings: 4

Ingredients

- 2 cups low-fat Greek yogurt
- 2 peaches, sliced
- ¼ cup granola
- Honey for drizzling (optional)

Directions

1. In serving glasses, layer Greek yogurt and sliced peaches.
2. Top each parfait with granola and a drizzle of honey if desired.
3. Serve immediately or chill in the refrigerator until ready to serve.

Nutrition Facts (per serving)

- Calories: 150
- Fat: 2g
- Saturated Fat: 0g
- Cholesterol: 10mg
- Sodium: 45mg

- Carbohydrate: 22g
- Fiber: 2g
- Sugar: 18g
- Protein: 12g
- Calcium: 150mg
- Potassium: 300mg

Berry Gelatin Cups

Prep Time: 10 mins (plus chilling time)

Total Time: 4 hrs 10 mins

Servings: 4

Ingredients

- 2 cups mixed berries (strawberries, blueberries, raspberries)
- 1 packet unflavored gelatin
- 2 cups boiling water
- 2 tablespoons honey

Directions

1. Place mixed berries evenly into serving cups.
2. In a bowl, dissolve the gelatin in boiling water. Stir in honey until well combined.
3. Pour the gelatin mixture over the berries in the serving cups.
4. Refrigerate until set, about 4 hours.
5. Serve chilled, enjoying the natural sweetness of the berries.

Nutrition Facts (per serving)

- Calories: 100
- Fat: 0g
- Saturated Fat: 0g
- Cholesterol: 0mg
- Sodium: 40mg

- Carbohydrate: 24g
- Fiber: 2g
- Sugar: 20g
- Protein: 2g
- Calcium: 20mg
- Potassium: 120mg

Coconut Mango Mousse

Prep Time: 15 mins (plus chilling time)

Total Time: 2 hrs 15 mins

Servings: 4

Ingredients

- 1 ripe mango, peeled and cubed
- 1 can (14 oz) coconut cream, chilled
- 2 tablespoons honey
- ½ teaspoon vanilla extract
- Fresh mint leaves for garnish

Directions

1. Puree the mango in a blender until smooth.
2. In a mixing bowl, whip the chilled coconut cream until it forms soft peaks. Gently fold in the mango puree, honey, and vanilla extract until well combined.
3. Spoon the mousse into serving dishes and refrigerate for at least 2 hours, or until set.
4. Garnish with fresh mint leaves before serving.

Nutrition Facts (per serving)

- Calories: 280
- Fat: 22g
- Saturated Fat: 19g
- Cholesterol: 0mg
- Sodium: 15mg

- Carbohydrates: 22g
- Fiber: 2g
- Sugar: 20g
- Protein: 2g
- Calcium: 20mg
- Potassium: 260mg

Almond and Berry Crumble

Prep Time: 10 mins

Total Time: 30 mins

Servings: 4

Ingredients

- 2 cups mixed berries (fresh or frozen)
- 1 cup almond flour
- ¼ cup sliced almonds
- 2 tablespoons coconut oil, melted
- 2 tablespoons maple syrup
- ½ teaspoon cinnamon

Directions

1. Preheat oven to 375°F (190°C). Place berries in a baking dish.
2. In a bowl, mix almond flour, sliced almonds, melted coconut oil, maple syrup, and cinnamon until crumbly.
3. Sprinkle the almond mixture over the berries.
4. Bake for 20 minutes, or until the topping is golden and the berries are bubbly.
5. Serve warm, perhaps with a dollop of low-fat Greek yogurt.

Nutrition Facts (per serving)

- Calories: 280
- Fat: 18g

- Saturated Fat: 6g
- Cholesterol: 0mg
- Sodium: 10mg
- Carbohydrates: 24g
- Fiber: 6g
- Sugar: 16g
- Protein: 6g
- Calcium: 60mg
- Potassium: 200mg

Lemon Ricotta Cake

Prep Time: 15 mins

Total Time: 45 mins

Servings: 4

Ingredients

- 1 cup almond flour
- ½ cup ricotta cheese
- ¼ cup honey
- 2 eggs
- Zest of 1 lemon
- 1 teaspoon vanilla extract
- ½ teaspoon baking powder

Directions

1. Preheat oven to 350°F (175°C). Grease a small cake pan.
2. In a bowl, mix together almond flour, ricotta, honey, eggs, lemon zest, vanilla extract, and baking powder until smooth.
3. Pour the batter into the prepared cake pan.
4. Bake for 30 minutes, or until a toothpick inserted into the center comes out clean.
5. Let cool before serving, garnished with a sprinkle of powdered sugar if desired.

Nutrition Facts (per serving)

- Calories: 320
- Fat: 20g
- Saturated Fat: 6g
- Cholesterol: 110mg
- Sodium: 80mg
- Carbohydrates: 24g
- Fiber: 3g
- Sugar: 18g
- Protein: 12g
- Calcium: 150mg
- Potassium: 100mg

Chocolate Avocado Pudding

Prep Time: 10 mins

Total Time: 1 hr 10 mins (including chilling)

Servings: 4

Ingredients

- 2 ripe avocados, peeled and pitted
- ¼ cup cocoa powder
- ¼ cup honey or maple syrup
- ½ teaspoon vanilla extract
- Pinch of salt
- Fresh raspberries for garnish

Directions

1. In a blender, combine avocados, cocoa powder, honey (or maple syrup), vanilla extract, and a pinch of salt. Blend until smooth.
2. Divide the pudding into serving dishes and chill in the refrigerator for at least 1 hour.
3. Garnish with fresh raspberries before serving.

Nutrition Facts (per serving)
- Calories: 240
- Fat: 15g
- Saturated Fat: 2g
- Cholesterol: 0mg
- Sodium: 10mg
- Carbohydrates: 28g
- Fiber: 7g
- Sugar: 18g
- Protein: 3g
- Calcium: 20mg
- Potassium: 560mg

No-Bake Coconut Balls

Prep Time: 20 mins (plus chilling time)

Total Time: 1 hr 20 mins

Servings: 4

Ingredients

- 1 cup shredded coconut, unsweetened
- ½ cup almond flour
- ¼ cup coconut oil, melted
- ¼ cup maple syrup
- 1 teaspoon vanilla extract
- Pinch of salt

Directions

1. In a mixing bowl, combine shredded coconut, almond flour, melted coconut oil, maple syrup, vanilla extract, and a pinch of salt. Stir until well combined.
2. Roll the mixture into small balls, about 1 inch in diameter, and place them on a baking sheet lined with parchment paper.
3. Chill in the refrigerator for at least 1 hour, or until firm.
4. Serve chilled, stored in an airtight container in the refrigerator.

Nutrition Facts (per serving)
- Calories: 280
- Fat: 22g
- Saturated Fat: 18g
- Cholesterol: 0mg
- Sodium: 25mg
- Carbohydrates: 20g
- Fiber: 4g
- Sugar: 14g
- Protein: 3g
- Calcium: 40mg
- Potassium: 200mg

Baked Peach Crisp

Prep Time: 15 mins

Total Time: 45 mins

Servings: 4

Ingredients

- 4 ripe peaches, pitted and sliced
- 1 tablespoon lemon juice
- ½ cup rolled oats
- ¼ cup almond flour
- ¼ cup brown sugar
- ¼ cup unsalted butter, cold and cubed
- ½ teaspoon cinnamon
- Pinch of salt

Directions

1. Preheat oven to 350°F (175°C). Toss peach slices with lemon juice and arrange them in a baking dish.
2. In a bowl, mix rolled oats, almond flour, brown sugar, cinnamon, and a pinch of salt. Add cold butter and use your fingers to mix until crumbly.
3. Sprinkle the oat mixture evenly over the peaches.
4. Bake for 30 minutes, or until the topping is golden brown and the peaches are bubbly.
5. Serve warm, optionally with a scoop of low-fat vanilla ice cream or a dollop of whipped cream.

Nutrition Facts (per serving)

- Calories: 290
- Fat: 15g
- Saturated Fat: 8g
- Cholesterol: 30mg
- Sodium: 60mg
- Carbohydrates: 37g
- Fiber: 4g
- Sugar: 25g
- Protein: 4g
- Calcium: 40mg
- Potassium: 420mg

SMOOTHIE RECIPES

Blueberry Almond Smoothie

Prep Time: 5 mins

Total Time: 5 mins

Servings: 2

Ingredients

- 1 cup fresh blueberries
- 1 banana, sliced
- ½ cup unsweetened almond milk
- ¼ cup Greek yogurt
- 2 tablespoons almond butter
- 1 tablespoon honey (optional)
- Ice cubes

Directions

1. In a blender, combine blueberries, banana, almond milk, Greek yogurt, almond butter, and honey if using. Add a handful of ice cubes.
2. Blend on high until smooth and creamy.
3. Pour into glasses and serve immediately for a refreshing and nutritious smoothie.

Nutrition Facts (per serving)

- Calories: 220
- Fat: 11g
- Saturated Fat: 1g
- Cholesterol: 0mg
- Sodium: 80mg
- Carbohydrate: 27g
- Fiber: 4g
- Sugar: 18g (natural sugars from fruit; excludes optional honey)
- Protein: 7g
- Calcium: 150mg
- Potassium: 350mg

Spinach Avocado Smoothie

Prep Time: 5 mins

Total Time: 5 mins

Servings: 2

Ingredients

- 2 cups fresh spinach leaves
- 1 ripe avocado, peeled and pitted
- 1 cup unsweetened almond milk
- ½ cucumber, sliced
- Juice of 1 lime
- 1 tablespoon chia seeds
- Ice cubes

Directions

1. Place spinach, avocado, almond milk, cucumber, lime juice, and chia seeds in a blender. Add a handful of ice cubes.
2. Blend until smooth and creamy.
3. Serve immediately, enjoying the creamy texture and the health benefits of greens and healthy fats.

Nutrition Facts (per serving)

- Calories: 200
- Fat: 14g
- Saturated Fat: 2g
- Cholesterol: 0mg
- Sodium: 60mg
- Carbohydrate: 18g

- Fiber: 9g
- Sugar: 4g
- Protein: 5g
- Calcium: 180mg
- Potassium: 650mg

Strawberry Oatmeal Breakfast Smoothie

Prep Time: 5 mins

Total Time: 5 mins

Servings: 2

Ingredients

- 1 cup fresh strawberries
- ½ cup rolled oats
- 1 banana, sliced
- 1 cup low-fat milk or almond milk
- ½ teaspoon vanilla extract
- 1 tablespoon honey (optional)
- Ice cubes

Directions

1. Add strawberries, rolled oats, banana, milk, vanilla extract, and honey if using to a blender. Include a handful of ice cubes for a colder smoothie.
2. Blend on high until smooth and the oats are fully integrated.
3. Pour into glasses and serve for a filling and nutritious breakfast smoothie.

Nutrition Facts (per serving)

- Calories: 210
- Fat: 3g
- Saturated Fat: 0.5g
- Cholesterol: 5mg
- Sodium: 55mg
- Carbohydrate: 40g
- Fiber: 5g
- Sugar: 20g (natural sugars from fruit; excludes optional honey)
- Protein: 8g
- Calcium: 150mg
- Potassium: 450mg

Carrot Ginger Turmeric Smoothie

Prep Time: 5 mins

Total Time: 5 mins

Servings: 2

Ingredients

- 1 cup carrot juice
- 1 banana, sliced
- ½ teaspoon grated ginger
- ¼ teaspoon ground turmeric
- ½ cup orange juice
- Ice cubes

Directions

1. In a blender, combine carrot juice, banana, grated ginger, ground turmeric, and orange juice. Add a handful of ice cubes for a chilled smoothie.
2. Blend until smooth.
3. Serve immediately, taking advantage of the anti-inflammatory benefits of ginger and turmeric.

Nutrition Facts (per serving)

- Calories: 150
- Fat: 0.5g
- Saturated Fat: 0g

- Cholesterol: 0mg
- Sodium: 70mg
- Carbohydrate: 36g
- Fiber: 3g
- Sugar: 25g
- Protein: 2g
- Calcium: 20mg
- Potassium: 500mg

Mango Coconut Water Smoothie

Prep Time: 5 mins

Total Time: 5 mins

Servings: 2

Ingredients

- 1 cup mango chunks, fresh or frozen
- 1 cup coconut water
- Juice of ½ lime
- 1 tablespoon flaxseed meal
- Ice cubes

Directions

1. Place mango chunks, coconut water, lime juice, and flaxseed meal in a blender. Add a handful of ice cubes.
2. Blend on high until smooth and creamy.
3. Pour into glasses and serve immediately, enjoying the tropical flavors and hydrating properties of coconut water.

Nutrition Facts (per serving)

- Calories: 120
- Fat: 2g
- Saturated Fat: 0g
- Cholesterol: 0mg
- Sodium: 60mg
- Carbohydrate: 25g
- Fiber: 3g
- Sugar: 20g
- Protein: 2g
- Calcium: 30mg
- Potassium: 400mg

Banana Almond Smoothie

Prep Time: 5 mins

Total Time: 5 mins

Servings: 2

Ingredients

- 2 ripe bananas
- 1 cup almond milk, unsweetened
- 2 tablespoons almond butter
- ½ teaspoon vanilla extract
- Ice cubes (optional)

Directions

1. Combine bananas, almond milk, almond butter, and vanilla extract in a blender.
2. Add ice cubes to preference for a colder, thicker smoothie.
3. Blend until smooth and creamy.
4. Serve immediately for a refreshing and energizing drink.

Nutrition Facts (per serving)

- Calories: 280
- Fat: 15g
- Saturated Fat: 1.5g
- Cholesterol: 0mg
- Sodium: 80mg
- Carbohydrates: 36g
- Fiber: 6g

- Sugar: 18g
- Protein: 7g
- Calcium: 200mg
- Potassium: 600mg

Blueberry Spinach Smoothie

Prep Time: 5 mins

Total Time: 5 mins

Servings: 2

Ingredients

- 1 cup fresh spinach
- 1 cup blueberries, fresh or frozen
- 1 banana
- 1 cup almond milk, unsweetened
- 1 tablespoon flaxseeds

Directions

1. Place spinach, blueberries, banana, almond milk, and flaxseeds in a blender.
2. Blend until the mixture is smooth.
3. Serve immediately, enjoying the blend of antioxidants and fiber.

Nutrition Facts (per serving)

- Calories: 150
- Fat: 3g
- Saturated Fat: 0g
- Cholesterol: 0mg
- Sodium: 80mg
- Carbohydrates: 29g
- Fiber: 5g
- Sugar: 17g
- Protein: 3g
- Calcium: 150mg
- Potassium: 400mg

Strawberry Cucumber Smoothie

Prep Time: 5 mins

Total Time: 5 mins

Servings: 2

Ingredients

- 1 cup strawberries, fresh or frozen
- 1 small cucumber, peeled and sliced
- 1 cup coconut water
- Juice of ½ lime
- Mint leaves for garnish

Directions

1. Add strawberries, cucumber, coconut water, and lime juice to a blender.
2. Blend until smooth.
3. Pour into glasses and garnish with mint leaves.
4. Enjoy a hydrating and refreshing smoothie.

Nutrition Facts (per serving)

- Calories: 60
- Fat: 0g
- Saturated Fat: 0g
- Cholesterol: 0mg
- Sodium: 25mg
- Carbohydrates: 14g
- Fiber: 3g
- Sugar: 10g
- Protein: 1g
- Calcium: 40mg
- Potassium: 400mg

Peach Ginger Smoothie

Prep Time: 5 mins

Total Time: 5 mins

Servings: 2

Ingredients

- 2 peaches, sliced
- ½ inch piece of ginger, peeled
- 1 cup Greek yogurt, unsweetened
- 1 tablespoon honey (optional)
- Ice cubes

Directions

1. Place peaches, ginger, Greek yogurt, and honey (if using) in a blender.
2. Add ice cubes as desired.
3. Blend until smooth and creamy.
4. Serve immediately, savoring the spicy-sweet flavors.

Nutrition Facts (per serving)

- Calories: 120
- Fat: 0.5g
- Saturated Fat: 0g
- Cholesterol: 5mg
- Sodium: 35mg
- Carbohydrates: 24g
- Fiber: 2g
- Sugar: 20g (includes honey)
- Protein: 7g
- Calcium: 150mg
- Potassium: 350mg

Carrot Apple Ginger Smoothie

Prep Time: 5 mins

Total Time: 5 mins

Servings: 2

Ingredients

- 2 carrots, peeled and chopped
- 1 apple, cored and sliced
- ½ inch ginger, peeled
- 1 cup water or apple juice
- Ice cubes

Directions

1. Combine carrots, apple, ginger, and water/apple juice in a blender.
2. Add ice cubes to preference.
3. Blend until smooth.
4. Serve immediately, enjoying the invigorating and nutritious drink.

Nutrition Facts (per serving)

- Calories: 95
- Fat: 0.3g
- Saturated Fat: 0g
- Cholesterol: 0mg
- Sodium: 40mg
- Carbohydrates: 24g
- Fiber: 5g
- Sugar: 17g (less if using water)
- Protein: 1g
- Calcium: 30mg
- Potassium: 410mg

30-DAY MEAL PLAN

Day 1
- Breakfast: Oatmeal with Fresh Berries and Almonds
- Main Dish: Grilled Chicken with Herb Salad
- Snack: Cucumber and Hummus Bites
- Vegetables and Salad: Mixed Greens with Apple and Walnuts
- Soup and Stew: Chicken and Rice Soup
- Dessert: Baked Apples with Cinnamon
- Smoothie: Blueberry Almond Smoothie

Day 2
- Breakfast: Scrambled Eggs with Spinach and Feta
- Main Dish: Baked Salmon with Asparagus
- Snack: Apple Slices with Almond Butter
- Vegetables and Salad: Cucumber Tomato Salad
- Soup and Stew: Tomato Basil Soup
- Dessert: Vanilla Rice Pudding
- Smoothie: Spinach Avocado Smoothie

Day 3
- Breakfast: Cottage Cheese and Pineapple Bowl
- Main Dish: Quinoa Stuffed Bell Peppers
- Snack: Greek Yogurt with Honey and Walnuts
- Vegetables and Salad: Roasted Beet and Goat Cheese Salad
- Soup and Stew: Lentil Vegetable Stew
- Dessert: Peach Yogurt Parfait
- Smoothie: Strawberry Oatmeal Breakfast Smoothie

Day 4
- Breakfast: Quinoa Breakfast Porridge
- Main Dish: Turkey and Vegetable Skillet
- Snack: Carrot Sticks with Avocado Dip
- Vegetables and Salad: Carrot Slaw with Cranberries
- Soup and Stew: Butternut Squash Soup
- Dessert: Berry Gelatin Cups
- Smoothie: Carrot Ginger Turmeric Smoothie

Day 5
- Breakfast: Baked Avocado Eggs
- Main Dish: Lentil Soup with Spinach
- Snack: Baked Kale Chips
- Vegetables and Salad: Spinach and Strawberry Salad
- Soup and Stew: Carrot Ginger Soup

- Dessert: Coconut Mango Mousse
- Smoothie: Mango Coconut Water Smoothie

Day 6
- Breakfast: Greek Yogurt with Mixed Nuts and Honey
- Main Dish: Baked Cod with Roasted Vegetables
- Snack: Roasted Chickpeas
- Vegetables and Salad: Avocado and Tomato Salad
- Soup and Stew: Zucchini Basil Soup
- Dessert: Almond and Berry Crumble
- Smoothie: Banana Almond Smoothie

Day 7
- Breakfast: Chia Seed Pudding with Kiwi
- Main Dish: Turkey Meatballs in Tomato Sauce
- Snack: Zucchini Chips
- Vegetables and Salad: Broccoli and Cauliflower Salad
- Soup and Stew: Creamy Mushroom Soup
- Dessert: Lemon Ricotta Cake
- Smoothie: Blueberry Spinach Smoothie

Day 8
- Breakfast: Quinoa Breakfast Bowl
- Main Dish: Grilled Vegetable Platter
- Snack: Peanut Butter Banana Bites
- Vegetables and Salad: Cucumber Dill Salad
- Soup and Stew: Sweet Potato and Lentil Stew
- Dessert: Chocolate Avocado Pudding
- Smoothie: Strawberry Cucumber Smoothie

Day 9
- Breakfast: Berry Smoothie with Spinach
- Main Dish: Cauliflower Steak with Herb Sauce
- Snack: Cucumber Roll-Ups with Hummus
- Vegetables and Salad: Mixed Bean Salad
- Soup and Stew: Creamy Cauliflower Soup
- Dessert: No-Bake Coconut Balls
- Smoothie: Peach Ginger Smoothie

Day 10
- Breakfast: Oatmeal with Fresh Berries and Almonds
- Main Dish: Baked Tilapia with Lemon and Dill
- Snack: Avocado Toast with Cherry Tomatoes
- Vegetables and Salad: Shaved Brussels Sprout Salad
- Soup and Stew: Chicken Vegetable Soup

- Dessert: Baked Peach Crisp
- Smoothie: Carrot Apple Ginger Smoothie

Day 11
- Breakfast: Quinoa Breakfast Porridge
- Main Dish: Grilled Vegetable Platter
- Snack: Cucumber Roll-Ups with Hummus
- Vegetables and Salad: Mixed Bean Salad
- Soup and Stew: Creamy Mushroom Soup
- Dessert: Lemon Ricotta Cake
- Smoothie: Banana Almond Smoothie

Day 12
- Breakfast: Berry Smoothie with Spinach
- Main Dish: Baked Tilapia with Lemon and Dill
- Snack: Avocado Toast with Cherry Tomatoes
- Vegetables and Salad: Shaved Brussels Sprout Salad
- Soup and Stew: Sweet Potato and Lentil Stew
- Dessert: Chocolate Avocado Pudding
- Smoothie: Blueberry Spinach Smoothie

Day 13
- Breakfast: Oatmeal with Fresh Berries and Almonds
- Main Dish: Quinoa Stuffed Bell Peppers
- Snack: Greek Yogurt with Honey and Walnuts
- Vegetables and Salad: Cucumber Dill Salad
- Soup and Stew: Creamy Cauliflower Soup
- Dessert: No-Bake Coconut Balls
- Smoothie: Strawberry Cucumber Smoothie

Day 14
- Breakfast: Scrambled Eggs with Spinach and Feta
- Main Dish: Turkey and Vegetable Skillet
- Snack: Baked Kale Chips
- Vegetables and Salad: Avocado and Tomato Salad
- Soup and Stew: Chicken Vegetable Soup
- Dessert: Baked Peach Crisp
- Smoothie: Peach Ginger Smoothie

Day 15
- Breakfast: Avocado Toast with Poached Egg
- Main Dish: Lentil Soup with Spinach
- Snack: Roasted Chickpeas
- Vegetables and Salad: Broccoli and Cauliflower Salad
- Soup and Stew: Chicken and Rice Soup
- Dessert: Baked Apples with Cinnamon

- Smoothie: Carrot Apple Ginger Smoothie

Day 16
- Breakfast: Cottage Cheese and Pineapple Bowl
- Main Dish: Baked Cod with Roasted Vegetables
- Snack: Zucchini Chips
- Vegetables and Salad: Mixed Greens with Apple and Walnuts
- Soup and Stew: Tomato Basil Soup
- Dessert: Vanilla Rice Pudding
- Smoothie: Blueberry Almond Smoothie

Day 17
- Breakfast: Baked Avocado Eggs
- Main Dish: Turkey Meatballs in Tomato Sauce
- Snack: Peanut Butter Banana Bites
- Vegetables and Salad: Cucumber Tomato Salad
- Soup and Stew: Lentil Vegetable Stew
- Dessert: Peach Yogurt Parfait
- Smoothie: Spinach Avocado Smoothie

Day 18
- Breakfast: Greek Yogurt with Mixed Nuts and Honey
- Main Dish: Cauliflower Steak with Herb Sauce
- Snack: Cucumber and Hummus Bites
- Vegetables and Salad: Roasted Beet and Goat Cheese Salad
- Soup and Stew: Butternut Squash Soup
- Dessert: Berry Gelatin Cups
- Smoothie: Strawberry Oatmeal Breakfast Smoothie

Day 19
- Breakfast: Chia Seed Pudding with Kiwi
- Main Dish: Grilled Chicken with Herb Salad
- Snack: Apple Slices with Almond Butter
- Vegetables and Salad: Carrot Slaw with Cranberries
- Soup and Stew: Carrot Ginger Soup
- Dessert: Coconut Mango Mousse
- Smoothie: Carrot Ginger Turmeric Smoothie

Day 20
- Breakfast: Quinoa Breakfast Bowl
- Main Dish: Baked Salmon with Asparagus
- Snack: Greek Yogurt with Honey and Walnuts

- Vegetables and Salad: Spinach and Strawberry Salad
- Soup and Stew: Zucchini Basil Soup
- Dessert: Almond and Berry Crumble
- Smoothie: Mango Coconut Water Smoothie

Day 21

- Breakfast: Berry Smoothie with Spinach
- Main Dish: Quinoa Stuffed Bell Peppers
- Snack: Carrot Sticks with Avocado Dip
- Vegetables and Salad: Avocado and Tomato Salad
- Soup and Stew: Creamy Mushroom Soup
- Dessert: Lemon Ricotta Cake
- Smoothie: Banana Almond Smoothie

Day 22

- Breakfast: Oatmeal with Fresh Berries and Almonds
- Main Dish: Turkey and Vegetable Skillet
- Snack: Baked Kale Chips
- Vegetables and Salad: Broccoli and Cauliflower Salad
- Soup and Stew: Sweet Potato and Lentil Stew
- Dessert: Chocolate Avocado Pudding
- Smoothie: Blueberry Spinach Smoothie

Day 23

- Breakfast: Greek Yogurt with Mixed Nuts and Honey
- Main Dish: Lentil Soup with Spinach
- Snack: Greek Yogurt with Honey and Walnuts
- Vegetables and Salad: Roasted Beet and Goat Cheese Salad
- Soup and Stew: Butternut Squash Soup
- Dessert: Berry Gelatin Cups
- Smoothie: Strawberry Oatmeal Breakfast Smoothie

Day 24

- Breakfast: Chia Seed Pudding with Kiwi
- Main Dish: Baked Cod with Roasted Vegetables
- Snack: Carrot Sticks with Avocado Dip
- Vegetables and Salad: Carrot Slaw with Cranberries
- Soup and Stew: Carrot Ginger Soup
- Dessert: Coconut Mango Mousse
- Smoothie: Carrot Ginger Turmeric Smoothie

Day 25

- Breakfast: Quinoa Breakfast Bowl
- Main Dish: Turkey Meatballs in Tomato Sauce
- Snack: Baked Kale Chips

- Vegetables and Salad: Spinach and Strawberry Salad
- Soup and Stew: Zucchini Basil Soup
- Dessert: Almond and Berry Crumble
- Smoothie: Blueberry Almond Smoothie

Day 26

- Breakfast: Oatmeal with Fresh Berries and Almonds
- Main Dish: Grilled Chicken with Herb Salad
- Snack: Roasted Chickpeas
- Vegetables and Salad: Mixed Bean Salad
- Soup and Stew: Creamy Mushroom Soup
- Dessert: Lemon Ricotta Cake
- Smoothie: Mango Coconut Water Smoothie

Day 27

- Breakfast: Berry Smoothie with Spinach
- Main Dish: Cauliflower Steak with Herb Sauce
- Snack: Zucchini Chips
- Vegetables and Salad: Shaved Brussels Sprout Salad
- Soup and Stew: Sweet Potato and Lentil Stew
- Dessert: Chocolate Avocado Pudding
- Smoothie: Banana Almond Smoothie

Day 28

- Breakfast: Scrambled Eggs with Spinach and Feta
- Main Dish: Baked Tilapia with Lemon and Dill
- Snack: Peanut Butter Banana Bites
- Vegetables and Salad: Avocado and Tomato Salad
- Soup and Stew: Creamy Cauliflower Soup
- Dessert: No-Bake Coconut Balls
- Smoothie: Blueberry Spinach Smoothie

Day 29

- Breakfast: Avocado Toast with Poached Egg
- Main Dish: Baked Salmon with Asparagus
- Snack: Cucumber Roll-Ups with Hummus
- Vegetables and Salad: Broccoli and Cauliflower Salad
- Soup and Stew: Chicken Vegetable Soup
- Dessert: Baked Peach Crisp
- Smoothie: Strawberry Cucumber Smoothie

Day 30

- Breakfast: Cottage Cheese and Pineapple Bowl
- Main Dish: Quinoa Stuffed Bell Peppers

- Snack: Avocado Toast with Cherry Tomatoes
- Vegetables and Salad: Cucumber Dill Salad
- Soup and Stew: Chicken and Rice Soup
- Dessert: Baked Apples with Cinnamon
- Smoothie: Peach Ginger Smoothie

INTERACTIVE TOOLS TO MONITOR HIGH OXALATES

Oxalate Food Diary

Personal Information

- Name: _____
- Date: _____
- Health Goal: _____

Daily Food Intake Log

Meal Type	Food Item	Portion Size	Estimated Oxalate Content (mg)	Notes
Snack 1				
Lunch				
Snack 2				
Dinner				
Snack 3				

Daily Fluid Intake

Beverage Type	Amount (ml or oz)	Notes
Water		
Tea/Coffee		
Other		

Symptoms/Reactions Log

- Morning:

    - _____

- Afternoon:

    - _____

- Evening:

    - _____

- General Notes:

    - _____

Daily Reflection

- What went well today?

    - _____

- What could be improved?

    - _____

- Adjustments for tomorrow:

Oxalate Symptom Tracker

Personal Information

- **Name:** _____
- **Month/Year:** _____
- **Health Objective:** _____

Daily Symptom Log

Date	Symptoms Experienced	Severity (1-10)	Possible Trigger Foods	Notes

Weekly Summary

Week Ending	Most Common Symptoms	Average Severity	Foods to Avoid	Adjustments for Next Week

Notes and Observations

- Week 1:

    - _____

- Week 2:

    - _____

- Week 3:

    - _____

- Week 4:

    - _____

Monthly Reflection

- **Key Insights:**

    - _____

- **Dietary Adjustments Needed:**

    - _____

- **Next Steps/Action Plan:**

_____

_____

_____

_____

_____

Meal Planning Guide

Meal Planning Guide Worksheet

Personal Information

- Name: _____

- Week Of: _____

- Health Goals/Dietary Restrictions: _____

Weekly Meal Plan

Day	Breakfast	Snack 1	Lunch	Snack 2	Dinner	Notes
Monday						
Tuesday						

Wednesday						
Thursday						
Friday						
Saturday						
Sunday						

Grocery List

- **Fruits and Vegetables:**

    - _____

- **Proteins:**

    - _____

- **Dairy and Eggs:**

    - _____

- **Grains and Cereals:**

    - _____

- **Canned and Dry Goods:**

    - _____

- **Frozen Foods:**

    - _____

- **Beverages:**

    - _____

- **Miscellaneous:**

- _____

Prep Schedule

Day	Tasks
Monday	
Tuesday	
Wednesday	
Thursday	
Friday	
Saturday	
Sunday	

Notes/Reminders

- _____
- _____
- _____

Hydration Tracker

Creating a Hydration Tracker involves designing a layout that allows individuals to monitor their daily water intake, ensuring they meet their hydration goals. This tool is especially useful for maintaining general health, supporting kidney function, and aiding in the management of conditions that benefit from increased fluid intake. Below is a suggested format for the tracker, adaptable for digital use or printable for manual entries.

Hydration Tracker Worksheet

Personal Information

- **Name:** _____
- **Month/Year:** _____
- **Daily Water Intake Goal:** _____ liters/ounces

Daily Hydration Log

Date	Time	Amount (ml/oz)	Beverage Type	Notes

Weekly Summary

Week Ending	Total Intake (liters/ounces)	Goal Met (Y/N)	Notes

Notes and Observations

- **Week 1:**

    - _____

- **Week 2:**

    - _____

- **Week 3:**

    - _____

- **Week 4:**

    - _____

Monthly Reflection
- Key Insights:
    - _____
- Adjustments for Next Month:
    - _____

Medication and Supplement Monitor

Personal Information
- Name: _____
- Month/Year: _____
- Physician/Healthcare Provider: _____

Daily Medication and Supplement Log

Date	Medication/Supplement Name	Dosage	Time Taken	Notes

Weekly Summary

Week Ending	Missed Doses	Adjustments/Changes	Notes

Notes and Observations

- **Week 1:**

    - _____

- **Week 2:**

    - _____

- **Week 3:**

    - _____

- **Week 4:**

    - _____

Monthly Reflection

- **Key Insights:**

    - _____

- **Adjustments for Next Month:**

    - _____

- **Healthcare Provider Consultations:**

    - _____

Recipe Modification Worksheet

Personal Information

- **Name:** _____
- **Date:** _____
- **Dietary Goal/Requirement:** _____

Original Recipe Details

- **Recipe Name:** _____
- **Original Ingredients:**

    - _____
    - _____
    - _____

- **Preparation Steps:**

    - _____
    - _____
    - _____

Modification Plan

Original Ingredient	Suggested Substitute	Reason for Change	Adjusted Quantity

Adjusted Preparation Steps

- _____

- _____

- _____

Notes and Observations

- **Taste Test Results:**

    - _____

- **Texture and Consistency Adjustments:**

    - _____

Additional Modifications Needed:

- _____

Final Adjusted Recipe

- **Adjusted Ingredients:**

    - _____

    - _____

    - _____

- **Final Preparation Steps:**

    - _____

    - _____

    - _____

Nutrient Intake Chart

Personal Information

- **Name:** _____
- **Date:** _____
- **Dietary Goals:** _____

Daily Nutrient Intake Log

Nutrient	Recommended Daily Amount	Amount Consumed	Source(s) of Nutrient	Notes
Calories				
Protein (g)				
Carbohydrates (g)				
Dietary Fiber (g)				
Total Fat (g)				
Saturated Fat (g)				
Trans Fat (g)				
Cholesterol (mg)				
Sodium (mg)				
Potassium (mg)				
Vitamin D (µg)				
Calcium (mg)				
Iron (mg)				
Vitamin A (µg)				
Vitamin C (mg)				

Weekly Summary

Nutrient	Weekly Goal	Total Consumed	Average Daily Intake	Notes
Calories				
Protein (g)				
Carbohydrates (g)				
Dietary Fiber (g)				
Total Fat (g)				
Saturated Fat (g)				
Trans Fat (g)				
Cholesterol (mg)				
Sodium (mg)				
Potassium (mg)				
Vitamin D (µg)				
Calcium (mg)				
Iron (mg)				
Vitamin A (µg)				
Vitamin C (mg)				

Notes and Observations

- **Challenges Encountered:**

    - _____

- **Successful Strategies:**

    - _____

- **Adjustments for Next Week:**

    - _____

Eating Out Guide: Low-Oxalate Choices

Personal Information

- **Name:** _____
- **Date:** _____
- **Dietary Goal (Low-Oxalate):** _____

General Tips for Eating Out

- Choose grilled, baked, or steamed dishes over fried options.
- Opt for clear soups and broths; avoid cream-based soups.
- Request dressings and sauces on the side to control intake.
- Prioritize lean proteins like chicken, turkey, and fish.
- Select sides of steamed vegetables or salads with low-oxalate greens.
- Drink water or herbal teas instead of high-oxalate beverages.

Low-Oxalate Choices by Cuisine

Cuisine Type	Recommended Dishes	Dishes to Avoid	Notes
American	Grilled chicken, Baked potato, Garden salad (no spinach)	French fries, Spinach salad, Nuts and berries desserts	
Italian	Grilled seafood, Risotto, Caprese salad (moderate tomatoes)	Pasta with tomato-based sauces, Pizza with high-oxalate toppings	
Chinese	Steamed fish, Chicken and broccoli, White rice	Spinach dishes, Nuts in dishes, Brown rice	

| Mexican | Chicken fajitas (no tomato salsa), Rice and beans, Guacamole | Spinach enchiladas, Tomato salsa, Chocolate-based sauces | |
| Indian | Tandoori chicken, Lentil soup (check for spinach), Cucumber raita | Spinach curry, Tomato-based curries, Chutneys with high-oxalate ingredients | |

Restaurant Log

Date	Restaurant Name	Cuisine Type	Low-Oxalate Choices Made	Overall Experience	Notes

Reflection and Adjustments

- **Positive Experiences:**

    - _____

- **Challenges Encountered:**

    - _____

- **Adjustments for Future Dining Out:**

    - _____

Progress Reflection and Goal Setting Sheets

Progress Reflection and Goal Setting Sheets

Personal Information

- Name: _____
- Date: _____
- Primary Health/Dietary Goal: _____

Monthly Progress Reflection

Date	Achievements	Challenges	Insights Gained	Adjustments Needed

Weekly Goal Setting

Week Starting	Specific Goals	Action Steps	Resources Needed	Support System

Daily Check-In

Date	Goal Focus	Progress Notes	Mood/Well-being	Next Day's Focus

Quarterly Review

- **Key Achievements:**

    - _____

- **Persistent Challenges:**

    - _____

- **Long-Term Goal Adjustment:**

    - _____

- **New Skills/Learnings:**

    - _____

Goal Setting for Next Quarter

- **Primary Goal:**

    - _____

- **Milestones:**

    - _____

- **Potential Obstacles:**

    - _____

- **Support Needed:**

    - _____

CONCLUSION

Starting a journey toward better health, particularly by focusing on managing oxalate intake, is a noteworthy and vital path to take. The "Low Oxalate Food List, Cookbook, and Meal Plan for Seniors" isn't just a set of recipes and advice—it's a beacon of hope, highlighting the significance of making well-informed dietary decisions. As we age, recognizing the need to adjust our diet to meet our body's evolving requirements is crucial.

Grasping the nuances of oxalates and their effects on our health is a step towards empowerment. Armed with knowledge, we're positioned to make decisions that safeguard against health issues and boost our overall wellness. Your decision to use this guide marks a significant step. It's not solely about sidestepping certain foods; it's about adopting a lifestyle that values health, energy, and well-being.

The meal plans, recipes, and worksheets in this guide are your allies on this voyage. They're your navigation tools, helping you traverse the wide expanse of nutrition and wellness. Each recipe is created with both health and enjoyment in mind, ensuring that food remains a pleasure. The meal plans aim to add diversity and balance, making sure your diet is as engaging as it is nutritious.

The worksheets, from the Oxalate Food Diary to the Reflection and Goal Setting Sheets, bolster your active role in this health journey. They foster mindfulness and self-awareness, essential for enduring change. By monitoring your intake, symptoms, and progress, you're not merely following a plan; you're conversing with your body, understanding its signals, and meeting its needs.

Change, especially altering long-standing dietary habits, might seem intimidating. You might face moments of frustration or temptation. Yet, remember, every small step is progress towards a healthier you. Choosing a low-oxalate meal is a triumph, a pledge to your well-being.

If you feel overwhelmed or unsure, remember, you're in good company. This journey towards health is one many undertake, facing similar hurdles and celebrating alike successes. There's strength in this shared experience, in the collective knowledge of those who've walked this path before.

Consider this guide a foundation on which to build a diet and lifestyle that align with your health aspirations. Allow yourself the freedom to experiment, learn, and evolve. Health is a personal voyage, not a fixed endpoint. Approach this journey with curiosity, patience, and kindness towards yourself.

As you proceed, view each meal, each decision to adopt a low-oxalate diet, as a chance to nourish both body and soul. Taking care of yourself, selecting foods that heal and sustain, is an act of love—a testament to your self-worth and commitment to health.

In challenging moments, remember why you began. Whether it's managing a health condition, enhancing your well-being, or ensuring your golden years are enjoyed to the fullest, let this purpose guide you.

Moving forward with knowledge, tools, and recipes at your disposal, recall the words of Lao Tzu: "The journey of a thousand miles begins with a single step." Let each meal, each choice for a low-oxalate diet, be a step towards health. You hold the power to shape your health and future, one meal at a time.

May this guide accompany you on your journey, offering inspiration and a reminder of your strength and resilience. To your health, happiness, and the path ahead.

Dear Reader,

Thank you for embarking on this culinary journey with us through the pages of this book. We hope that it has served not just as a guide to a healthy cooking, but also as an inspiration for a joyful and healthy approach to food that complements your lifestyle and dietary needs.

Your feedback is invaluable to us. It not only celebrates our shared achievements but also lights the path for future improvements. We warmly invite you to share your thoughts and experiences with this cookbook. Did the recipes spark new ideas in your kitchen? Were the food lists and meal planning strategies helpful in managing your diet? Any favorite dishes or suggestions for what you'd like to see more of in future editions? Your honest review can help others in their decision to embark on a similar journey and enable us to enhance the value we provide in our next works.

Here's how you can leave a review on Amazon:

Log into your Amazon account: Navigate to Amazon.com and sign in with the account you used to purchase the book.

Find the book: You can easily locate the book by typing "Low Oxalate Diet Cookbook Meal Plan and Food List for seniors by Hilda M. Jacobs" into the search bar. Once you've found the book, click on its title to visit the product detail page.

Scroll to Customer Reviews: On the product detail page, scroll down until you reach the "Customer Reviews" section.

Write a review: Click on the button labeled "Write a customer review." Amazon will then guide you to a page where you can rate the book by selecting 1 to 5 stars, add a headline for your review, and write your thoughts and experiences in the text box provided.

Submit your review: After filling out your review, click the "Submit" button to share your feedback with the Amazon community.

Sharing your insights is more than just a review; it's a contribution to a community of readers seeking guidance and inspiration for managing diabetes through diet. We're deeply grateful for your time and effort in providing your feedback.

Warmest regards,

Hilda M. Jacobs

www.ingramcontent.com/pod-product-compliance
Lightning Source LLC
Chambersburg PA
CBHW062218220526
45471CB00009B/3258